WHAT YOU MUST KNOW ABOUT

LIVER DISEASE

A PRACTICAL GUIDE TO USING CONVENTIONAL AND COMPLEMENTARY TREATMENTS

RICH SNYDER, DO

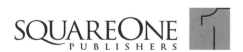

SQUAREONE
PUBLISHERS

EDITOR: Caroline Smith
COVER DESIGNER: Jeannie Tudor
TYPESETTER: Gary A. Rosenberg

Square One Publishers
115 Herricks Road
Garden City Park, NY 11040
(516) 535-2010 • (877) 900-BOOK
www.squareonepublishers.com

Library of Congress Cataloging-in-Publication Data

Names: Snyder, Rich, author.
Title: What you must know about liver disease : a practical guide to using conventional
    and complementary treatments / Rich Snyder, DO.
Description: Garden City Park, NY : Square One Publishers, [2016] | Includes
    bibliographical references and index.
Identifiers: LCCN 2016015603 (print) | LCCN 2016015856 (ebook) | ISBN 9780757004049
    (pbk. : alk. paper) | ISBN 9780757054044
Subjects: LCSH: Liver—Diseases—Popular works. | Liver—Diseases—Alternative
    treatment—Popular works.
Classification: LCC RC846 .S69 2016 (print) | LCC RC846 (ebook) | DDC 616.3/62—dc23
LC record available at https://lccn.loc.gov/2016015603

10   9   8   7   6   5   4   3   2   1

Contents

This book is dedicated to all individuals and their families who may be struggling with liver disease or other chronic illness. We acknowledge your courage, your fortitude, and your heart.

Acknowledgments

I would like to thank Rudy Shur, who has been a constant source of encouragement concerning this book and previous books we have done together. I would like to also acknowledge Caroline Smith. She is a truly phenomenal editor and it was a pleasure to work with her on this book.

I would like to finally acknowledge my mother, Nancy Snyder, RN, who truly encompasses the healing spirit and whose empathy and compassion know no bounds.

A Word About Gender

In an effort to avoid awkward phrasing within sentences, it is our publishing style to alternate the use of male and female pronouns according to chapter. Therefore, when referring to a "third-person" adult, child, healthcare provider, or caregiver, odd-numbered chapters will use female pronouns, while even-numbered chapters will use male, to give acknowledgment to people of both genders.

Introduction

According to the American Liver Foundation, approximately thirty million people in the United States have been diagnosed with liver disease. That means one out of every ten people is affected by a disease such as hepatitis, cirrhosis, or liver cancer. And although your liver is essential to sustaining a healthy life because it performs many important processes in the body, it is often overlooked.

The scary aspect about liver diseases is that you can have one for a long time without being aware that something is wrong. It is only when the condition has dramatically worsened that you begin to experience its symptoms and understand the effect it can have on your health. That is why it is so important to know about the risk factors and initial signs of liver diseases. The earlier you can catch a liver problem, the better your outcome will be.

What You Must Know About Liver Disease will provide you with the fundamental information you need to know to gain insight into how well your liver is functioning. You will be able to identify your risk factors for liver disease, as well as the important steps you can take to prevent one from occurring in the first place. If you have already been diagnosed with a liver disease, it is vital to understand your treatment and management options, which will also be discussed in this book.

The goal of this book is to provide you with the basics of liver disease. Because liver disease can be complex, understanding the basics is crucial for you to effectively work with your doctor and other health care providers in formulating a treatment plan. This is meant to be a "beginner-level book" that gives you the information you need in an easy-to-read and understandable format.

Through reading this book, you will gain an understanding not only of the dietary and lifestyle changes that you can make to improve your liver health, but also of the clinical side of various disorders so that you can effectively work with your health care provider to create a personalized treatment plan.

The book is divided into two parts to provide you with an integrated view of the treatment of liver diseases. You first gain an understanding of the most common liver diseases and the treatment strategies available. Then, you review the complementary and alternative treatments that can be used to improve this organ's health.

Part One, "An Introduction to Liver Disease," provides you with the fundamentals of the liver and its diseases. You learn about where this important organ is located, the basic functions it performs, and its role in your overall health. You review the most common conditions, as well as the various means that doctors use to define, diagnose, and treat them. The causes of liver disease will be explained, as well. I tell you about how to get the most out of your office visits when talking to your family doctor, a liver specialist, or to a team of liver transplant coordinators. You also gain a clear understanding of commonly ordered blood tests that physicians will use to better evaluate your liver function, and what they mean.

Part Two, titled "Complementary Treatment Approaches and Lifestyle Changes," places the focus on prevention and treatment, especially on complementary and alternative methods that you can utilize to improve your liver function. You will learn about ways in which you can develop a detox plan for your liver, without feeling hungry or exhausted.

An important chapter in this section discusses the dietary changes you will need to make to create a "liver-based nutrition plan." As obesity and poor diet are major causes of liver disease in industrialized countries, this chapter is significant in its prevention. The nutrition plan that you adopt today can only be beneficial to your health in the future. In addition to dietary and lifestyle changes, in Part Two you learn about natural supplements and herbs, as well as an exercise plan, that you can add to enhance your treatment regimen.

Whether you have the risk factors for liver disease (but have not been diagnosed with one) or you have been living with a liver disease for years, this book arms you with the tools and information that you need to give yourself the best outcome possible. The knowledge that you gain from this book will allow you to be your own advocate for your health care. Let's get reading!

PART ONE

An Introduction to Liver Disease

I f you have been diagnosed with a liver disease, you may feel over-whelmed. You may not know how you came to develop your liver disease, or know where to begin when it comes to treating it. You may not have given much thought to your liver before your diagnosis. Well, the fact is you are not alone! Many people are unaware of just how fundamental the liver is to maintaining total body health. The first part of this book consists of seven chapters, which serve to provide you the basic information about the most common liver ailments—including their symptoms, their causes, and the common treatments used to help. It will also include explanations of the many health care professionals who are involved in testing for and treating it.

The goal of Chapter 1 is to enable you to understand the importance of the liver and the many functions it performs. These include processing and metabolizing all of the substances you consume, clotting the blood, filtering out toxins, producing proteins, and more.

In Chapter 2, you will learn more about liver disorders and how detrimental to your wellbeing an unhealthy liver can be. You will read about the differences between acute and chronic conditions. I will also talk about the most common diagnostic tests that your doctor will initially order and use to evaluate your condition. These are the tests that will confirm if any liver diseases are present or not.

Chapter 3 talks about specific liver illnesses in more depth. Several of the most common conditions, including hepatitis and cirrhosis, are discussed here. For each of these diseases, I have provided information about common signs and symptoms, risk factors, causes, possible complications, diagnostic methods, treatments, and prognosis. This information can serve as a basic guide for you and can be especially helpful when talking to your doctor. This chapter serves as a foundation for the rest of the book; it provides with you a basic and necessary vocabulary so that you can better understand the many nuances of liver disease.

Chapter 4 expands upon the complications of liver diseases. Although the liver is unwell, it is often not the only body part that is affected. Important organs such as the kidneys, the heart, and the brain can be harmed by liver disease. In this chapter, you will learn about what signs and symptoms to be aware of that can indicate a liver ailment is spreading to other parts of the body.

In Chapter 5, I talk about medications. This includes the treatments for various conditions, but also the common prescription and over-the-counter drugs that can actually further damage the liver. It is important to distinguish between when medication can improve your health and your quality of life, and when medication may be too much for your liver to handle. This chapter also explains how to manage your medication, as the options available to you may become overwhelming.

Over the course of your treatment, you may meet with several doctors and other health care professionals. What is the difference between a gastroenterologist and a hepatologist? What about a nutritionist and a dietitian? Can seeing an integrative health care provider be helpful? The roles of these doctors are identified and explained in Chapter 6. This chapter will also give you tips on making the most of your doctor's appointments; a list of questions to ask your health care providers is included. Being an active participant and an effective communicator during your treatment is very important.

Finally, in Chapter 7, I discuss liver transplants. Liver transplants are very successful treatments, but unfortunately, they can be difficult to obtain. This chapter explains the process of gaining a spot on the transplant waiting list; it then tells you what to expect before, during, and after the surgery. Just as the roles of the health care professionals are explained in Chapter 6, Chapter 7 provides a look at the members of the liver transplant team.

You may have a lot of questions when you are first diagnosed with a liver disease; it is my hope that with the first part of this book, these questions will be answered in a way that empowers you to make the best decisions about your health.

1

Your Liver and You

Your liver is one of the largest and most important organs in your body. It performs many vital and life-preserving functions and is the body's "processor," serving to clean the blood of toxins and provide the body with nutrients. The liver works conjointly with several other organs, including the gallbladder, intestines, and the kidneys, to maintain a healthy body. The significance of the liver is often overlooked until one is diagnosed with a liver disease, and by then, it may be too late to reverse the damage. Given the prevalence of liver disease, it is important to do all that you can to optimize your liver health and preserve its function. As a doctor of internal medicine, I often see people who are unaware either that they have a liver disease or are at serious risk of developing one. This book is dedicated to informing you with all you need to know about the liver and liver health. In this chapter, you will learn not only about where the liver is located, but also about the important and diverse functions that it performs.

WHERE IS THE LIVER LOCATED?

The liver resides on the upper right-hand side of your abdomen, underneath the diaphragm and protected by your rib cage. It sits next to the stomach and just above the gallbladder. The liver works together with these organs to digest food, metabolize nutrients, detoxify the body, and other important functions. (Refer to a diagram of the liver shown in Figure 1.1.)

Try and recall the last time you went to see your doctor or health care provider for a physical. When the doctor finished listening to your heart and lungs, she likely asked you to lie down on the exam table so that she

5

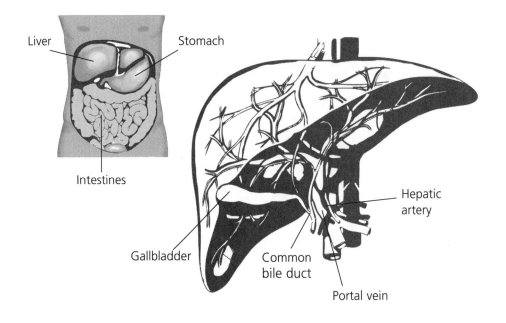

Figure 1.1. A diagram of the liver.

could examine your abdomen. A common method that doctors use to examine the liver is *palpation* (*pal-pay-shun*), or placing their hands (clean and hopefully not cold!) around the area underneath your right rib cage. They are trying to see if they can feel the bottom-most aspect of the liver, also called the "liver edge." Your doctor should *not* be able to palpate, or feel, the edge of the liver below the rib cage. If she does, this indicates that there may be a problem with the liver. If she can feel the liver edge, this may be a sign that you have an enlarged liver, or *hepatomegaly* (*hep-atto-meg-a-lee*). This will require further evaluation.

When your doctor presses her hand against the part of your abdomen where your liver is located, you should not feel any pain or discomfort in that area. If you do experience tenderness, this may indicate a problem with either the liver or the gallbladder. The gallbladder is an organ that sits just below the liver and is involved with many of the liver's functions, especially digestion.

In an average-sized individual, a healthy liver weighs approximately forty-eight ounces (three pounds). The liver usually measures just under three inches in length for women and a little over four inches in length in men. A smaller than average liver can suggest the presence of *cirrhosis* (*sir-row-siss*), a chronic liver disease. A liver larger than the aforementioned sizes may suggest *hepatitis* (*hep-a-tie-tiss*), an acute inflammation. You can read more about these conditions in Chapters 2 and 3.

ANATOMY OF THE LIVER

In later chapters, I will reference some parts of the liver's anatomy, including the bile ducts, the nerve fibers, and the vessels that carry blood to and from the liver. This section will give a brief overview of these components. Knowing which specific part of the liver is affected by disease is important for prompt diagnosis, treatment, and recovery.

The liver is split into the right lobe and the left lobe. These two main lobes contain thousands of lobules, which all connect to small ducts. Together, these ducts form the common hepatic duct. This duct transports *bile* (*bye-ull*) from the liver to the gallbladder and intestines. Bile aids the body in digesting food. (See page 9 for more information about the liver's role in digestion).

The entire liver is enclosed in a thin layer of tissue. The liver itself does not contain nerve fibers and cannot feel pain; however, this surrounding tissue does have nerve fibers. These nerve fibers become irritated if the tissue is stretched by a tumor or inflammation. This can cause abdominal pain, which is often an initial sign of a problem in the liver.

Blood is supplied to the liver through two distinct blood vessels: the hepatic artery and the portal vein. The hepatic artery distributes blood to the liver, as well as to other gastrointestinal organs, such as the stomach, gallbladder, and pancreas. The portal vein also delivers blood to the liver; this blood comes from the spleen and the gastrointestinal tract, and therefore carries an abundance of nutrients. The portal vein is the source for about 75 percent of the liver's nutrients, while the hepatic artery supplies the majority of the liver's oxygen.

The liver is normally a "low-pressure" system. If you were to measure the pressure in the liver and compare it with the rest of the body, you would find that the liver's pressure is lower. It is this lower pressure that keeps the blood and other body fluids flowing through the liver normally. Increased pressure in the portal vein can be a sign of cirrhosis, as we will discuss in Chapter 2.

Liver Regeneration

The liver is the only organ in the body that has the extraordinary ability to regenerate itself. It can fully regenerate up to 75 percent of damaged tissue in about a month, assuming there are no further complications (such as excessive drinking) during that time. Studies of liver regeneration in mice have shown that cells in the liver called *hepatocytes* replicate and restructure themselves, in response to signals from hormones, proteins, and other signaling pathways. Most of the functions that the liver performs are not compromised during regeneration. Because of the amount of damaging toxins and chemicals that the liver is exposed to, regeneration is an important process in maintaining the liver's health. It is also essential for patients who need to have part of their liver removed due to tumor, disease, or other damage. Liver generation is what makes it possible for a living person to donate a part of her liver to somebody else. (See Chapter 7 for information about liver transplants.)

WHAT DOES THE LIVER DO?

Your liver carries out many important functions; its primary job is to be the body's "processor." The liver processes, or *metabolizes* (*met-taa-bo-lies-es*), practically everything you ingest, including the food that you eat and the medications that you are prescribed. The liver processes blood that flows through it from the stomach and intestines. This blood contains nutrients from digested food. The nutrients make their "first stop" in the liver, since breakdown products from digestion need to be separated before the nutrients can be transported to other parts of the body. Beverages that you consume, including alcohol, are also metabolized in the liver. Additionally, the liver processes many of the body's hormones.

Some substances that we ingest, most notably alcohol, can be toxic to the liver. Often, what damages the liver is the excessive consumption of products (such as medications) that are tolerable in normal amounts. (See Chapter 5 for more information about how medications can affect the liver.) Usually, the liver removes toxic products from the body through waste or converts the toxic products into harmless materials. However, over time, the liver can become diseased and damaged as a consequence of being "overloaded" by excess alcohol or other substances.

Below, we will go into the liver's most vital functions. These functions are carried out by cells called *hepatocytes* (*hep-ah-toe-sites*), which make up about 75 percent of the cells in the liver. In addition to these functions, the hepatocytes can also help the liver regenerate tissue (see the inset "Liver Regeneration" on page 8).

Clots the Blood

In addition to being the body's "processor," the liver is responsible for clotting your blood. This is one of the most vital functions of the liver. If you cut yourself, the liver is responsible for the production of *coagulation factors,* or "clotting factors," that prevent you from excessively bleeding or bruising. The liver can do this partially because it stores and processes vitamin K, which is necessary for clotting. If your liver is diseased, its ability to properly clot your blood can be affected. In the setting of a very diseased liver, even taking a vitamin K supplement will not help clot the blood, as the liver will be unable to fully process it. This increases the risk of increased bleeding and bruising.

Detoxifies the Body

The liver plays a large role in detoxifying the body. The enzymes and pathways in the liver are not only responsible for processing hormones and medications, but also for metabolizing the toxins that we are exposed to on a daily basis. These toxins can come from pesticides and chemicals in the foods you consume, or heavy metals in your water and surrounding environment. Medications can have byproducts, also referred to as toxic *metabolites* (*met-tab-o-lytes*). The liver is responsible for processing all of these harmful materials. If you think about the toxic load that the liver is exposed to on a daily basis, you will realize that your liver does a lot of work. That's why it is important to pay attention to the environment around you, as well as the purity of the foods that you consume and the amount of medication you ingest. They all play an important role in helping you maintain your liver health. (See Chapter 8 for more information about liver detoxification.)

Digests Food

The liver works together with the gallbladder to help digest food. The liver produces a substance called bile. Bile is made up of water, bile salts, cholesterol, and *bilirubin* (*billy-ruben*), a brownish-yellow substance that is produced when the liver processes old red blood cells. An excess of bile can cause gallstones (see inset "Gallstones" below), which can be an indicator of a problem in the liver. After bile is produced, it travels through various passageways, or "ducts," (called bile ducts) until it reaches the gallbladder, where it is stored until needed. When you eat, the digested food in your small intestine stimulates the release of bile from the gallbladder. The bile helps your intestine further break down and absorb the fats from the meal you recently ate. The fats produce energy for the body to use.

In addition to fats, the liver also metabolizes carbohydrates from the foods and beverages you consume. For example, the liver regulates the level of sugar in your blood; if your blood sugar level is high, the liver will take sugar out of the blood and store it as glycogen (a complex sugar). If your blood sugar level is low, the liver releases sugar into the bloodstream after breaking down the stored glycogen. The liver also stores vita-

Gallstones

Some people may experience gallstones (lumps in the gallbladder). These lumps can cause a "gallstone attack," where the patients may suffer intense pain in their upper abdomen, between their shoulder blades, or below their right shoulder, as well as nausea and/or vomiting. Gallstones are formed from excess cholesterol that is contained in bile. They can also be caused by an overabundance of bile in the gallbladder (due to infrequent emptying of the gallbladder). Gallstones are effectively treated by surgical removal of the gallbladder, which has few to no negative effects for the majority of patients.

While a poor diet is a risk factor in developing gallstones, no clear relationship has been established between the two. Cirrhosis of the liver, which you will read more about in Chapter 2, is another risk factor. Having a healthy liver may not completely eliminate the risk of developing gallstones, but the steps you can take to prevent liver disease—including the implementation of a healthy diet and exercise—are certainly helpful in lessening the risk of gallstones as well. We will go over complementary treatments and lifestyle changes to improve liver health in Part Two of this book.

mins and minerals, such as iron, and releases them into the body when levels become low.

The liver is important for handling the protein that you consume on a daily basis. It helps break down and process the protein efficiently so that it can be used by the body. This is done by converting the amino acids (the "building blocks" of protein) in foods so that they can produce energy. This process creates a toxic byproduct called *ammonia,* which the liver converts into a less harmful substance and eliminates from the body. As you may have guessed, when the liver is diseased, its ability to process protein is affected. This will be an important fact to keep in mind when we discuss nutritional and dietary considerations for liver disease in Part Two of this book.

As an additional benefit, bile has antibacterial properties and can kill harmful bacteria that may be present in food.

Makes Cholesterol

The liver is responsible for the body's production of cholesterol. In fact, cholesterol is one of the "main ingredients" in bile. Cholesterol is often perceived as being "bad"—but cholesterol can have its benefits, too. The liver produces high-density lipoprotein (HDL, or "good") cholesterol, which absorbs excess cholesterol and transports it to the liver for removal. The liver also produces low-density lipoprotein (LDL, or "bad") cholesterol, which carries cholesterol and fat from the liver to the rest of the body. Cholesterol is the basic building block for many hormones that your body makes, including anabolic hormones (used in muscle repair) and reproductive hormones. However, if your level of cholesterol is too high, it can cause hard, fatty deposits in your arteries—giving cholesterol its "bad" reputation.

Millions of people are prescribed statin medications, which are used to reduce high cholesterol and high triglyceride levels. These medications act on the liver to inhibit the production of cholesterol. As you'll read in Chapter 5, statin medications can have a negative effect on the liver.

Produces Proteins

The liver is responsible for producing many important proteins. Examples of these include *albumin* (*owl-byu-min*) and *ferritin* (*ferret-in*). Albumin is the predominant protein in the blood, making up about 50 percent of plasma proteins. Albumin binds to and neutralizes toxic materials, preventing them from harming your body. It also transports substances such as calcium and magnesium to other parts of the body.

One of albumin's main functions is maintaining the body's fluid compartments; it prevents fluid from leaking out of the bloodstream. Think about it like this: Your body has several spaces, including "blood spaces" and "water spaces." The "blood spaces" are where the blood flows, such as veins and arteries. The "water spaces" are tissues in the body in which water is stored. Albumin helps to keep these important spaces separate. One consequence of low albumin levels is that fluid can cross spaces it normally wouldn't—for example, fluid can cross from the tissue into the blood vessels. When fluid moves to a space it should not normally be in, it is called *edema* (*uh-deema*). Edema usually presents as swelling in the legs and ankles. Edema or excess fluid that is caused by low albumin levels is one of the first signs of liver disease.

Another important protein that can be affected by a liver ailment is ferritin. Ferritin is responsible for the storage of iron. Iron helps create red blood cells, which carry oxygen to the rest of the body. However, free iron (iron that is unbound to a protein) is toxic to cells. Ferritin is vital because it stores and releases iron in a non-toxic form. The liver has a way of "sensing" which proteins and minerals the body needs at a certain time. For example, if your body needs to recover from a rapid blood loss, ferritin in the liver will release iron. When the liver becomes diseased or damaged, its ability to maintain this balance is reduced.

If you have liver disease, the liver's ability to properly produce certain proteins can become compromised. Albumin and ferritin are sometimes referred to as "acute phase reactants," as their levels respond to inflammation. For example, if you have a chronic illness or are experiencing inflammation, the liver produces less albumin. Conversely, some chronic illnesses can cause the liver to produce more ferritin. If a routine blood test shows a very high ferritin level (i.e., a ferritin level in the thousands of nanograms per milliliter, or ng/mL), it signals to your doctor that there is an acute or chronic illness affecting your body. The cause of the elevated ferritin level will need to be further investigated.

Regulates Immune Function

Your liver and your small and large intestines are the body's "center of immunity"—they do much more than digest food! Together, the liver and the intestines regulate the body's immune system. In addition to albumin and ferritin, the liver is responsible for the production of *antibodies*, which are proteins that fight infection. Cells in the liver called *Kupffer cells* clean the large amounts of blood that pass through the liver. These cells remove bacteria, fungi, parasites, and other harmful materials.

Your small and large intestines are made up of a large ecosystem of bacteria called *microflora*. Research on the microflora's role in the intestines is still being conducted. However, so far, the research has demonstrated that these flora (along with the liver) are very important for regulating the body's immune system. As you will read, healthy intestines and a healthy liver are key to maintaining a strong immune system.

SUMMARY

The liver is an essential organ to the body and performs several important functions, including clotting the blood, protecting the body from toxins, producing bile for digestion, processing nutrients from food, producing proteins and cholesterol, and regulating the immune system. As you can see, these processes and many others are affected when the liver becomes damaged. When the liver is not performing optimally, tissue in the body can die from lack of nutrients and toxins can enter the bloodstream, leading to serious consequences. Disease prevention is key for optimizing liver health, as we will discuss in the upcoming chapters.

2

A General Overview of Liver Disease

I n Chapter 1, you learned about the many functions the liver performs on a daily basis. "Liver disease" refers to any medical condition, toxin, or other substance or material that affects the liver's ability to properly carry out these important functions. In this chapter, I will define what liver disease is. There are two basic characterizations of liver disease, acute and chronic; these will be discussed in this chapter. Although dozens of conditions have been identified, most fall into one of these two categories. I will also explain the common signs and symptoms of liver disease and go over the ways health care professionals establish whether a condition is present. The common tests that doctors use to determine a diagnosis will be presented. This chapter will familiarize you with the most basic concepts of liver disease. Specific information about various illnesses will be discussed in further detail in Chapter 3.

WHAT IS LIVER DISEASE?

"Liver disease" is a broad term that describes any condition that damages the liver and prevents it from successfully functioning. There are dozens of conditions—genetic, viral, or otherwise—that fall under the category of liver disease. The most common ones are hepatitis, cirrhosis, and non-alcoholic fatty liver disease (NAFLD). As we will discuss below, liver conditions can be defined as *acute* or *chronic*. Acute liver disease has a rapid onset, with symptoms occurring over the course of a few days or weeks. Chronic liver disease is ongoing (sometimes for years) and develops at a slower pace. A problem with the liver is considered "chronic" after being present for six months.

Acute Liver Disease

As mentioned above, a liver disease is considered acute if it lasts less than six months and develops quickly. The most common illness that can cause an acute inflammation of the liver is *hepatitis* (*hep-uh-titus*). There are five types of hepatitis; these are simply called A, B, C, D, and E. We will go into detail about these diseases in Chapter 3, but below is a brief description of each:

- **Hepatitis A (HAV).** Hepatitis A is normally mild and those infected usually make a full recovery. It is transmitted through human waste via contaminated water, food, or sometimes through sexual contact with an infected person. There are vaccines available for HAV.

- **Hepatitis B (HBV).** Hepatitis B is the most common type worldwide. It normally lasts about six months, but can become a chronic disease and can lead to cirrhosis or liver cancer. It is transmitted by infected mothers to their children through birth. It can also be transmitted through sharing needles or other equipment that can spread bodily fluids, including contaminated medical equipment. There are vaccines available for HBV.

- **Hepatitis C (HCV).** Similarly to hepatitis B, hepatitis C is transmitted through exposure to contaminated blood, often through needles. Hepatitis C is the most common type in the United States. Hepatitis C is likely to become chronic. Many infected people experience no symptoms and do not realize they have it. There are no vaccinations available for HCV.

- **Hepatitis D (HDV).** Hepatitis D only occurs in individuals who have already been infected with HBV. Having both types conjointly can lead to a more dangerous illness, such as cirrhosis. HBV vaccines can prevent HDV.

- **Hepatitis E (HEV).** Similarly to hepatitis A, hepatitis E is transmitted through ingesting contaminated water or food. It is more common in developing nations. There are vaccines for HEV, but they are not widely available.

You may have also heard of hepatitis F and hepatitis G. Hepatitis F is a suspected type of hepatitis, but no virus has been found or confirmed for it. Hepatitis G was first identified in the mid-1990s. The virus has not yet been demonstrated to lead to acute or chronic hepatitis. It affects about 2 percent of the world's population and almost always co-occurs with hepatitis A, B, or C; HGV infection on its own is rare. The viruses that cause hepatitis G are related to the viruses that cause hepatitis C. Not much is known about hepatitis F or G, but they are not thought to be immediately dangerous or life-threatening.

There are many possible causes behind acute hepatitis. Hepatitis types A through E are caused by certain viruses. Another significant cause of acute hepatitis is excessive alcohol consumption, referred to as *alcoholic hepatitis.* (Refer to Chapter 3 for further discussion of specific causes.) The cause of the acute hepatitis is a factor in determining how long it will take for the liver to recover. For example, a virus called the *Epstein-Barr virus* (EBV) causes fever, sore throat, and fatigue. You may be familiar with it if you have ever had *mononucleosis* (more commonly known as the "kissing disease"), because EBV can cause mononucleosis. Very rarely, EBV can also affect the liver and cause acute hepatitis. Using this example, it may take a few weeks for someone with acute hepatitis due to EBV to recover.

In contrast, heavy alcohol consumption often elevates an acute hepatitis into a chronic disease, such as cirrhosis or even liver failure. In some cases, immediately stopping alcohol ingestion may eventually reverse the liver damage; in other cases, the patient may be unable to recover from the liver disease.

Three different scenarios can occur when someone is diagnosed with acute hepatitis: His liver can recover from the acute injury or inflammatory process and heal within a few weeks or a few months (depending on the nature of the hepatitis-inducing event); the liver can get worse very quickly (an uncommon phenomenon called *fulminant hepatitis*); or, he can develop a chronic liver problem, as we discuss below.

Chronic Liver Disease

A chronic disease is one that lasts longer than six months. The onset of a chronic liver disease is not as apparent and quick as an acute illness; often, a patient who is chronically sick shows no obvious symptoms. Over time, an acute liver problem can develop into a chronic liver problem. For example, some forms of acute hepatitis, such as hepatitis C, can become *chronic hepatitis.* Another chronic liver disease is *cirrhosis* (*sir-row-siss*), which will be discussed further in the next section.

Whether or not someone will develop a chronic liver disease often depends on the initial cause of the liver ailment. Some people are born with a congenital disorder (a hereditary condition) that affects the liver, such as *hemochromatosis* (an excess of iron in the body) or *Wilson's disease* (an excess of copper in the body). Congenital disorders such as these are considered to be chronic. Meanwhile, repeated injury to the liver (such as heavy drinking in an individual who already has acute liver disease) increases the risk of developing chronic cirrhosis.

In some cases, chronic liver disease can remain stable for months or years; symptoms may be mild or not noticeable at all. The liver will still be able to perform all of its many functions that you read about in Chapter 1. The most common example of this is a condition called *fatty liver disease*, which is an accumulation of fat in the cells of the liver. This can take place over the course of several years. (Fatty liver disease will be discussed in more detail in Chapter 3.) Just because symptoms are not obvious does not mean that treatment is optional—it is important to understand that a chronic liver problem can worsen over time.

Factors that determine whether or not the liver disease will worsen over time include the nature of the liver disease itself; the overall health of the liver and individual; and other superimposing acute illnesses or injuries. If an individual has poor nutrition, has other chronic medical conditions that can affect his overall health (e.g., diabetes), or exhibits lifestyle practices that can be toxic to the liver or the entire body (such as smoking and drinking), these factors can increase the risk of the individual having a liver issue that becomes worse over time. These issues put together can have a serious impact on liver health.

Cirrhosis

The most prevalent chronic liver disease is cirrhosis. Cirrhosis is the scarring of the liver. It reflects an ongoing process of chronic liver damage and is often not discovered or diagnosed until it has significantly progressed. It is important to make this fact clear: Having a chronic liver disease does not necessarily mean you have cirrhosis. However, if you are diagnosed with cirrhosis, it does mean that you have had a significant and chronic process affecting your liver.

If you were to use a microscope to look at hepatocytes—the cells of the liver—that have cirrhosis, you would see a significant amount of scarring in those cells. The more scarring that is visible, the more damage that has been done to the liver. Here is a way to think about scarring of the liver: If you were to cut yourself, you would have an acute injury to the skin and over time, a scar would form. Scars on the skin are permanent; they do not usually disappear or dissolve over time. If you have repeated cuts or injuries to your skin, you will see more scars. This is akin to what is happening to a cirrhotic (*sir-row-tic*) liver; a significant amount of scar tissue is forming on the liver over time.

Because cirrhosis is usually not reversible, it is important to investigate *why* the liver is becoming damaged. As previously mentioned, heavy drinking can lead to cirrhosis. Chronic hepatitis B or C can develop into cirrhosis due to long-term inflammation and damage. Many times, it is an acute event (like an infection or heavy bleeding) that stresses the body and overtaxes an already compromised liver. For example, if somebody already has a chronic liver disease, repeated acute illnesses or unhealthy habits can push the liver "over the edge" and increase the risk of that person developing cirrhosis. The reverse is also true: Having cirrhosis can lessen the body's ability to recover should it contract an acute illness (see inset below).

Cirrhosis:
It's Not Just a Liver Problem

If you have cirrhosis, it is not just the liver that is impacted. A study from the peer-reviewed journal *Chest* assessed the degree to which cirrhosis affects the survival of critically ill patients. They did this by examining the results from hospital discharges from 1995 to 1999. The authors found that cirrhosis is a risk factor for certain issues, including the development of a serious infection called *sepsis* that affects the whole body; acute breathing problems in the hospitalized setting; and mortality due to infection and acute respiratory failure. (Cirrhosis is consistently included in the top fifteen causes of mortality in the United States.) Additional complications of cirrhosis include malnutrition and an excess of toxins in the blood and brain, due to the liver's diminished ability to act as the body's filter and processor. It is not just the liver that is affected if you have cirrhosis; the study found that having cirrhosis can significantly impair your ability to recover from a serious infection or sepsis in a hospitalized setting. As this book emphasizes, the liver plays an important role in immunity.

The degree to which the liver can overcome an acute event is determined by how much "liver reserve" (how much healthy liver that is left, or
residual liver function) that you have. When a liver has diminished func-
tional reserve, it does not take much to overwhelm the liver. An example of
this kind of scenario is when somebody with cirrhosis is admitted to the
hospital after developing pneumonia. The acute pneumonia stresses the
body, particularly the liver and kidneys. Over time, it can be very difficult
for an already vulnerable liver to handle an acute "stress load" like this.

WHAT ARE THE SIGNS AND SYMPTOMS OF LIVER DISEASE?

There are different signs and symptoms that can be attributed to liver disease. While acute hepatitis, chronic liver disease, and cirrhosis sometimes
share the same symptoms, there are also significant differences between
these conditions. Below, I will list each of these conditions and the symptoms you should pay attention to.

Hepatitis and Acute Liver Disease

Many of the initial symptoms of hepatitis can be non-specific and attributed to a myriad of other causes. Examples of these include fatigue, weakness, weight loss, muscle and joint aches, decreased appetite, fever, and
lethargy. (See "Other Symptoms" on page 22.) As you can see, these symptoms are commonly found in a number of medical conditions. It is these
broad symptoms that are often the motivation for someone to visit his
doctor and undergo some testing. This testing can determine if there is
something wrong with the liver and if further evaluation is needed.

Because these initial symptoms of hepatitis can be non-specific, it is
important to not only pay attention to the nature of the acute symptoms,
but also their duration. Many viral illnesses or "twenty-four-hour bugs"
tend to persist for only a short time. If you are experiencing any or all of
the above symptoms, and they have lasted a week or more, it is important
to call your health care provider as soon as possible, as you likely need to
be further evaluated.

There are two other symptoms that may indicate that you have an
acute liver problem:

- **Jaundice** (*john-diss*). Jaundice refers to a yellowing of the skin. Jaundice also refers to yellowing of the eyes, which can sometimes precede

the yellowing of the skin (depending on the underlying condition). This condition is relatively specific to liver disease, especially acute hepatitis. It is caused by an excess of bilirubin (waste product) in the blood, which builds up because the liver is too diseased to remove it in the proper amounts.

- **Abdominal pain.** Sometimes, the process that is causing the acute hepatitis can cause the liver to become enlarged due to the inflammation. As you read in Chapter 1, the liver is encased in a capsule. When that capsule experiences swelling, its nerve fibers can become irritated. This in turn causes abdominal pain. The pain is usually located in the upper aspect of the abdomen, under the last rib on the right-hand side. If a doctor were to press on that area, it can cause intense pain and discomfort if the liver is "inflamed."

Cirrhosis

The most distinctive symptoms of cirrhosis are related to the level of pressure in the liver. As mentioned in Chapter 1, the liver is considered a "low-pressure" system. In the setting of cirrhosis, however, the scar tissue that develops in the cells can cause the pressure in the liver to build up over time. The "blood pressures" in the liver are often referred to as "portal pressures." This is because there is a buildup of pressure in the portal vein (and often the hepatic artery as well). When the pressures in the liver rise to a level greater than 35 millimeters of mercury (mmHg), it is called *portal hypertension*. The buildup of pressure in the liver can lead to fluid buildup, which presents in the following symptoms:

- **Ascites** (*a-cite-tees*). Ascites is the buildup of fluid in the abdominal cavity, and is most commonly caused by advanced liver disease or cirrhosis. It is a consequence of portal hypertension. Ascites can cause a "pregnant" appearance and weight gain. Other symptoms include difficulty breathing, indigestion, and abdominal pressure. Often, this fluid needs to be removed by a process called *paracentesis* (*para-sen-tee-siss*). This is usually done by either a liver specialist (*hepatologist* or *gastroenterologist*) or a physician called an *interventional radiologist* (IR doctor for short). For many with advanced liver conditions, this is a process that needs to be done on a regular basis, sometimes even weekly. Your doctor may prescribe certain medications that not only reduce the pressure in the liver, but also try to decrease the rate of fluid buildup in the abdomen. You can read more about these medications in Chapter 5.

- **Edema.** Edema (mentioned in Chapter 1) is the buildup of fluid in the legs and ankles. Signs of edema can include difficulty in putting shoes or pants on. You may get on a scale and notice that you have gained weight. Sometimes the edema can be "pitting," meaning that if you were to place your thumb or forefinger in the front of your leg below your knee and press on the skin, you would be able to make an indentation in the leg. As you will read in Chapter 5, common types of prescription medications that a physician will order to treat edema are called *diuretics* (*die-ur-ehtics*). Note that there can be many other causes of edema, including heart disease, congestive heart failure, and kidney disease. Sometimes these conditions may coexist with liver disease. Edema can also occur in acute or chronic hepatitis if the hepatitis is severe enough.

Other signs of cirrhosis can include symptoms that are also found in acute hepatitis, such as decreased appetite, fatigue, jaundice, lethargy, muscle and joint aches, weakness, and weight loss.

Other Symptoms

Although these are less common than the previously mentioned symptoms, there are other symptoms of liver disease that you should be aware of.

Sometimes there can be a difference in the color of your urine if acute or chronic liver disease is present. In Chapter 1, you read that there are many pathways and enzymes in the liver that are responsible for metabolizing and processing substances. In acute hepatitis and advanced cirrhosis, these pathways do not work as well, causing bilirubin to build up. When the bilirubin is unable to be further processed by the liver, it is then eliminated in the urine and can change the urine to an orange or almost dark brown hue. (Blood in the urine can also occur—see the inset "Can Liver Disease Cause Blood in the Urine?" on page 23.) Elevated bilirubin levels can be seen in both acute hepatitis and chronic cirrhosis.

Excessive bleeding or bruising can indicate a problem with the liver. A liver that is damaged has a decreased ability to produce the proteins that are needed for blood clotting.

Can Liver Disease Cause Blood in the Urine?

You may recall from Chapter 1 that one of the liver's main functions is to clot the blood. If you cut yourself, for example, the liver makes clotting factors that help to stabilize the acute injury and help prevent you from bleeding excessively. One of the consequences of a malfunctioning liver is increased risk of bruising and bleeding, as your liver is not able to make the clotting factors as effectively as it used to. You may notice that you bruise easier and that it takes longer for a bleeding injury, like a cut, to stop bleeding.

A question that is often asked in clinical practice is, "Can liver disease cause blood to appear in the urine?" The answer is yes and no. Yes, if your liver has difficulty clotting your blood, then this can be a cause of blood in the urine. But generally, having liver disease is not the sole cause of blood in the urine. If this is happening to you, it needs to be investigated further. Your health care provider or a specialist called a *urologist* can help in this

Cognitive issues, such as confusion, an inability to concentrate, forgetfulness, fatigue, and a change in sleeping patterns, can be present in both acute and chronic illnesses. When liver function deteriorates, there is an accumulation of waste and a decrease in the level of oxygen in the blood. The toxins that build up in the blood can spread to the brain, leading to these symptoms. In particular, the buildup of ammonia in the body (due to advanced liver disease) can precipitate a condition called *hepatic encephalopathy*, which is characterized by confusion and lethargy.

For similar reasons, unexplained vomiting and/or severely decreased appetite can be an indicator of liver damage. The excessive waste products in the body can cause digestive discomfort, nausea, and a loss of appetite, as well.

HOW YOUR DOCTOR DETERMINES IF LIVER DISEASE IS PRESENT

The signs and symptoms discussed in the prior sections often will be the first clues to your doctor that liver disease may be present. To confirm that the problem definitely lies in the liver, the doctor may need to order blood work or perform a series of tests that evaluate how well the liver is carrying out its functions.

Looking at Liver-Specific Blood Work

In this section, we will discuss general blood work that your doctor might order to determine if you have a liver problem. The blood testing discussed in this section only informs your doctor if there is a *general* liver problem. Often, your doctor will need to order further blood work to try and determine the specific cause of your liver problem. Please refer to Chapter 3 for information on specific conditions and the lab work that your doctor would order to evaluate for those conditions.

If your doctor has a suspicion that you have a liver problem, the test that he will most likely order first is the "liver function tests" (LFT), also referred to in some labs as the "hepatic (liver) function panel." There are five different components to the liver function tests: albumin, alkaline phosphatase, alanine aminotransferase (ALT), aspartate aminotransferase (AST), and total bilirubin. Your doctor not only looks at the value of each one, but also evaluates all of them together to get a picture of what may be going on with your liver. Let's take a look at each one in more detail.

Albumin

Albumin is a protein that is made by the liver. It is one of the most abundant proteins in the human body and is the body's major storage protein. The level of albumin in your body is thought to be reflective of your nutritional status. Be aware that there are many things that can affect an albumin level; a normal albumin level is usually around 4 grams per deciliter (g/dl). It is also referred to by doctors as an "acute phase reactant," meaning that its level reflects that there is an illness in the body. Many different medical conditions (acute or chronic) can decrease the level of albumin in the body. One major reason is that inflammation or illness in other parts of the body causes the liver to decrease the production of certain proteins (including albumin), while increasing the production of others (including antibodies to fight off infection, for example). Liver disease can be a cause of low albumin levels as well; in addition to an inflammatory "inhibition of albumin production," the more advanced the illness, the less capable is the liver's ability to produce proteins that the body requires (see the inset "The Liver Function Tests and Cirrhosis" on page 25). Other conditions that can lower the albumin levels are kidney disease (albumin can be lost through the urine; this is called *proteinuria*), malabsorption, and malnutrition.

The Liver Function Tests and Cirrhosis

Remember that cirrhosis refers to scarring of the liver. Keep in mind that a person may have cirrhosis, but have normal results in the liver function tests. This is because the liver cells are so scarred due to cirrhosis that they are not able to generate an increase in enzyme levels. The alanine aminotransferase (ALT) and aspartate aminotransferase (AST) levels may be normal, as may the alkaline phosphatase. Often the albumin and total protein levels will be low in someone with cirrhosis. This means that the context in which the labs are obtained is important: A "normal" test may not mean that the liver is okay, because cirrhosis may still be present. There are other blood tests and imaging studies that your doctor can order if there is a suspicion of cirrhosis. These are discussed further in the rest of this chapter.

Alkaline Phosphatase

This is a protein that can be elevated in some forms of liver disease. Like total bilirubin (see below), issues concerning the biliary system (such as gallstones) can raise levels of this blood test.

Alanine Aminotransferase (ALT) and Aspartate Aminotransferase (AST)

These are enzymes that are specific to the liver. They can be elevated in any type of acute liver damage (e.g., in acute hepatitis). The degree and quantity of elevation can often help the doctor figure out the cause of the liver dysfunction.

Total Bilirubin

Bilirubin can be elevated in certain forms of liver disease. It can also be elevated in other conditions that affect the "biliary system," including acute gallbladder inflammation, biliary stones, or biliary colic.

Other Liver Blood Tests

The following tests are commonly ordered by physicians to evaluate more specific aspects of the blood that can help diagnose a liver problem. Some of this blood work can be evaluated from the liver function tests above; for others, more blood needs to be drawn.

Basic Metabolic Panel

This is a routine blood test that your doctor will initially order in addition to the complete blood count (see below) and the liver function tests. The basic metabolic panel looks at electrolytes (such as sodium), measurements of kidney function (including creatinine level), and glucose and carbon dioxide levels. Low glucose and carbon dioxide levels can be indicative of advanced liver disease. One of the liver's important functions is to generate glucose when the body's level is too low; if the basic metabolic panel shows a low glucose level, it can signify that the liver is not functioning properly.

Carbon Dioxide (CO2) Level

This is a test that is part of a basic blood chemistry panel that your doctor might order. A normal level is approximately 22 to 24 milliequivalents per liter (meq/L). A lower value than this may mean that *acidosis* is present. Acidosis is an excess of acid in the blood. This problem occurs more often in very advanced cases of liver disease. One important aspect of the liver is that it regulates your body's acid-base balance; the liver is responsible for producing the bicarbonate (think baking soda) that the body needs to maintain *homeostasis,* or total body balance. By taking a look at the carbon dioxide level on routine lab work, health providers can monitor the liver's ability to maintain this acid-base homeostasis.

Complete Blood Count (CBC)

This is a routine test that your doctor will often order in conjunction with the liver function tests. Included in this test are the white cell count, hemoglobin count (the oxygen-carrying molecules in red blood cells), hematocrit (the volume percentage of red blood cells), and platelet count. Many individuals with chronic conditions may have anemia (a condition in which there are not enough red blood cells in the body), lower-than-normal white cell count, and/or low platelets. There are multiple possible causes of this in someone who has liver disease: If the spleen is enlarged (see page 28), many white cells and platelets can become "confiscated" in the spleen. In addition, substances such as alcohol can be toxic to the bone marrow and cause decreased production of white cells and platelets, as well as increase the risk of developing anemia.

Gamma-glutamyl Transferase (GGT)

GGT is an enzyme specific to the liver that is elevated in all types of liver disease. This is a test that is commonly ordered if your health care provider wants to confirm that you do, in fact, have an affliction of the liver.

Prothrombin Time (PT)

Recall from Chapter 1 that one of the many functions of the liver is clotting the blood. The PT is a blood test that can help determine how well your blood is clotting. Results for this test are given as an international normalized ratio (INR). A normal reference range for this value is between 0.8 and 1.1. If your number is higher than this, it may mean that there is a clotting problem with your liver. It is a very commonly ordered blood test that can be used to assess the "synthetic function of the liver."

Total Protein

This component of the test tells the doctor the levels of all of the major proteins of the body (these are proteins other than albumin). The doctor uses the degree of elevation from normal levels to determine if you are dealing with an acute process or a chronic process. For example, if an acute inflammatory process such as hepatitis is taking place, the body goes into "fight mode" to try and deal with the illness. This can entail increases in the ferritin and total protein levels, but a decrease in the albumin level. (As mentioned above, the albumin level is often low when you have an acute inflammatory illness.) The total protein level is raised because of the production of *immunoglobulins* (*imm-you-know-glob-u-linz*). Immunoglobulins (also referred to as antibodies) are larger-sized proteins whose production is increased during an illness. Conversely, in advanced cases of liver disease, such as cirrhosis, the liver may not be able to produce proteins to the levels that the body requires. You can see how the combination of the albumin and total protein counts can paint a picture for the doctor to get a better sense of what is going on with the liver.

Uric Acid

Uric acid is produced when the body breaks down purines, which are substances that occur naturally in the body and in certain foods. The test for uric acid is commonly ordered for the evaluation of gout (a form of arthritis), but several studies have demonstrated its importance in the context of liver sicknesses as well. A 2010 study by the peer-reviewed jour-

nal *Hepatology* looked to see if there was any correlation between an elevated uric acid level and the presence of either abnormal liver function
tests or the development of cirrhosis. The study investigators reviewed the
records of over 5,000 patients over a period of twelve years. The authors
concluded that the high uric acid levels were not only associated with the
development of elevated liver function tests (including GGT, mentioned
on page 27), but were also associated with the development of cirrhosis.

Looking at the Liver Directly

In addition to blood work, there are certain imaging studies that can give
your doctor a sense of what is going on. These include a liver ultrasound
and a computerized tomography (CT) scan. An ultrasound uses sound
waves that harmlessly bounce off of the internal organs to form an accurate image. A CT scan usually involves the patient drinking a solution
and injecting a dye. X-rays are taken of the patient's internal organs; the
dye helps create a cross-sectional image. If acute hepatitis is suspected,
your doctor will often order an ultrasound; if the acute hepatitis is present, the ultrasound will show an enlarged liver, also referred to as
hepatomegaly (*hep-at-toe-meg-uh-lee*). On the other hand, if cirrhosis is present, the ultrasound will show a small, shrunken liver. The liver scarring
can also be seen on the ultrasound.

Sometimes, a magnetic resonance imaging (MRI) machine is used to
look at potential damage to the liver. As the name suggests, an MRI machine
uses magnets and radio waves to create an image of internal organs.

Another common radiologic study that can be ordered is a specialized
type of nuclear medicine study called a "liver-spleen scan." This is a
nuclear medicine type of study in which a special kind of signal or tracer
moves through the blood in the liver and spleen. This type of study can
be used to help evaluate if liver disease is present. This test requires that
a medical professional place an intravenous (IV) line in your arm, as the
tracer needs to be given via the IV. The liver-spleen scan looks for signs
of ailments like cirrhosis and *hepatosplenomegaly* (*hep-at-toe-splenno-meg-a-
lee*), which is the enlargement of both the spleen and the liver.
Hepatosplenomegaly can occur as a result of portal hypertension, which
is a symptom of cirrhosis (as you read on page 21). When blood pressure
in the portal vein system increases, less blood can flow through the
splenic vein. The blood builds up and causes the spleen to grow in size.
Likewise, the pressure and congestion cause the liver to enlarge.

If your doctor suspects that cirrhosis is present, he may order an abdominal ultrasound or CT scan to evaluate not only the liver, but the spleen as well. (The ultrasound is preferred as it is less expensive and more accurate for looking at the liver.)

Looking at the Tissue Directly

Sometimes, despite blood work and other investigative studies, your doctor may still need to perform a test called a liver *biopsy* to see what is going on. In a liver biopsy, a small sample of tissue is taken by either a liver specialist (such as a gastroenterologist) or an interventional radiologist (IR). A physician specialist called a *pathologist* (*path-all-uh-jist*) then examines the tissue under a microscope for changes in the liver that can signify liver damage. Liver biopsies are important for determining not only the cause of the liver dysfunction, but also the degree of damage that has been done. For example, under the microscope, the pathologist can see the degree of inflammation in the liver as well as the extent of scarring, or *fibrosis*, that is present. This is important in painting a true picture of your overall liver health.

Note that a liver biopsy is an invasive procedure, as the tissue from the liver is taken from the blood vessels, from a needle through the skin, or from abdominal surgery. An alternative procedure, called a Fibroscan, is a non-invasive ultrasound-based study that can help determine if cirrhosis is present or not. Another name for this type of study is *ultrasound elastrography* (*e-last-tog-ra-fee*). It can help evaluate the stiffness of the liver. In one study, the results of this scan were compared to the biopsy results in looking at patients with viral hepatitis. The results demonstrated that the Fibroscan is nearly as reliable as a biopsy in measuring the extent of fibrosis in the liver.

SUMMARY

Most liver diseases can be characterized as acute (lasting less than six months, with a rapid onset) or chronic (lasting six months or more, with slow development). In this chapter, I discussed acute viral hepatitis and cirrhosis, a chronic condition. These conditions, and several others of note, will be discussed further in the next chapter.

The initial signs that you may have a liver problem are nonspecific and include fatigue, weakness, weight loss, muscle and joint aches, decreased appetite, fever, and lethargy. Other symptoms that are more specific to the liver are jaundice, ascites, and edema. Do not ignore these symptoms; seek medical attention if they do not go away. Your doctor initially will want to do a thorough medical history and physical examination to check for the signs and symptoms mentioned in this chapter. Further evaluation of liver disease includes blood testing, an imaging test such as an ultrasound or a CT scan, and sometimes a biopsy to figure out what is wrong.

3

A Closer Look at Liver Disease

The term "liver disease" can encompass dozens of conditions. In the previous chapter, I discussed the differences between acute and chronic liver disease. I reviewed hepatitis, a common presentation of acute liver disease, and cirrhosis, an example of a chronic illness. In this chapter, I will go more into detail about these conditions; you will also read about more conditions that can affect the liver. We will cover each condition's symptoms, causes, possible complications, diagnostic tests, treatments, and prognosis. Many of these conditions can overlap; it is often a combination of multiple "insults" to the liver (e.g., fatty liver combined with chronic acetaminophen and alcohol use) that affect it over the long term.

VIRAL HEPATITIS

As I briefly discussed in the previous chapter, hepatitis is an inflammation of the liver. It is most often caused by a fatty liver (which can lead to hepatitis) or by excessive drinking (alcoholic hepatitis). In this section, I discuss viral hepatitis, which is another common cause of liver inflammation. The five types of viral hepatitis are hepatitis A, B, C, D, and E. Of these, hepatitis B and C are very prevalent in the United States and in industrialized countries. Here, we will take a more in-depth look at each type.

HEPATITIS A

Hepatitis A is caused by the virus of the same name. It is an infection of the liver that causes inflammation and flu-like symptoms, such as fatigue and fever. Hepatitis A is very contagious and is more common in the developing world.

Signs and Symptoms

Many of the symptoms of acute hepatitis A are similar to those of acute hepatitis that you read about in Chapter 2. Symptoms usually present themselves two to six weeks after initial exposure to the hepatitis A virus. These symptoms can include:

- Decreased appetite
- Jaundice
- Diarrhea
- Weakness
- Generalized fatigue
- Weight loss

While many of these symptoms pose little danger, they can last for up to several months. If these symptoms persist for longer than a week, see a doctor.

Risk Factors

Hepatitis A is generally spread from contaminated feces. The following factors can increase the chance of someone contracting the virus:

- Having HIV or a clotting disorder (e.g., hemophilia).
- Having sexual contact with someone who has hepatitis A.
- Living in an area with poor sanitation, contaminated drinking water, and/or where hepatitis A vaccinations are not widely available.
- Using drugs that involve needles. (This mode of transmission is much more common for hepatitis B and C; however, it has been recognized as a potential mode of transmission for hepatitis A as well.)
- Working in a medical center.

Causes

Hepatitis A is transmitted by the "fecal-oral route." This means that the primary way to contract this condition is to eat food that is infected with the hepatitis A virus. Undercooked food, food that has been improperly prepared, or food prepared by an infected person who did not wash her hands are the main sources of this virus. There have been several case reports that linked undercooked shellfish or shellfish cooked in contaminated water as modes of transmission.

Hepatitis A is more prevalent in developing countries than it is in industrialized countries. In fact, many children in developing countries have become infected with hepatitis A and have developed antibodies to it. In the majority of cases, once the virus has been contracted, the infected person becomes resistant to any future exposure.

Note that while eating contaminated food is the most common form of transmission, this virus can also be transmitted directly from one person to another. This often occurs when the same people occupy a close space, especially one where there is poor sanitation or poor hygienic practices. Hepatitis A outbreaks occurring simultaneously in the same household have been recorded.

Possible Complications

Generally, hepatitis A poses no risk of complications. It usually is contained within the liver and heals on its own within six months. However, complications can occasionally occur. These include:

Cholestasis

This is an uncommon condition in which bile is not removed through the gallbladder (as it normally is) and builds up in the liver. It normally resolves by itself, but in a small percentage of individuals, it can cause long-lasting jaundice, diarrhea, and fever.

Liver Failure

On very rare occasions, hepatitis A can cause liver failure. This is more likely if the infected person's immune system is severely compromised and/or the patient has a pre-existing liver disease, such as cirrhosis. Signs of liver failure include excessive bleeding, fever, edema (fluid buildup in the legs), and ascites (fluid buildup in the abdomen). In the case of liver failure, a transplant may be necessary.

Relapse

In most cases, those who have contracted hepatitis A become immune to future attacks because of antibodies that remain in the body for life. However, in some cases, hepatitis A can recur with the same symptoms as the initial outbreak.

Diagnosis

A physical exam may be carried out by your doctor to check for hepatitis A. This involves the doctor pressing her hand on your lower right rib cage, feeling for an enlarged, protruding, or tender liver. As mentioned in Chapter 2, blood may be drawn for testing as well. These tests look for raised IgM and IgG antibodies. These antibodies are produced by the body to fight the hepatitis A virus. If the IgM antibodies are positive, this means that you are dealing with an acute infection. After your body has been infected by the hepatitis A virus, your immune system produces IgG antibodies; these antibodies will persist for years after the infection has gone. In most cases, the presence of these antibodies will provide immunity from re-infection. The physical exam and blood test together can confirm a diagnosis of hepatitis A.

Treatment

The treatment consists mainly of supportive care; there is no specific antidote for this condition. As previously mentioned, hepatitis A usually disappears on its own within six months of onset. In the majority of cases, those infected with hepatitis A become immune to it afterward, thanks to the IgG antibodies that remain in the blood.

Getting enough rest and avoiding alcohol and drugs (including over-the-counter medications, such as Tylenol, that are harmful to the liver—see Chapter 5) are recommended. One of the most important aspects of treatment is preventing the contraction of the virus in the first place. This can be as simple as washing your hands. Always wash your hands if you come into contact with another person's bodily fluids. If you are traveling to a high-risk area, be aware of what and where you eat; avoid undercooked meat and fish, and drink bottled water whenever possible. It is recommended that individuals who are traveling to high-risk areas obtain the hepatitis A vaccine. The vaccine is also recommended for individuals who are in close contact with a significant other, friend, or family member who has been diagnosed with hepatitis A.

Prognosis

Unlike other forms of hepatitis, hepatitis A does not usually cause chronic liver disease. The majority of the time, it is a condition that is limited to the liver and completely recovers. While in a few cases it can progress to fulminant (sudden and severe) liver failure, this is felt to be the exception rather than the rule.

HEPATITIS B

Hepatitis B is the most common form of viral hepatitis worldwide. It is caused by a DNA virus that is spread through bodily fluids. It can cause both acute and chronic hepatitis. (Refer back to Chapter 2 for more general information concerning both acute and chronic hepatitis.)

Signs and Symptoms

The symptoms of hepatitis B normally occur one to four months after the virus's initial onset. These symptoms may include:

- Dark urine
- Jaundice
- Decreased appetite
- Nausea and vomiting
- Fatigue
- Pain in the abdomen
- Fever

Risk Factors

The risk of developing hepatitis B increases for those who live in an area with a high rate of infection; those who share needles or other personal items that exchange bodily fluids; and those who have sexual contact with an infected person. Because risk factors for the development of hepatitis B include coming into contact with blood or other bodily fluids from a person infected with the virus, health care workers are at significant risk for acquiring hepatitis B. This is because they are often exposed to infected blood and needles.

The risk is also increased for those who have received organ or blood donations, especially before 1987; although blood banks have screened for exposure to the hepatitis B virus since 1987, these tests by themselves are unable to determine if the donor has actually contracted the disease.

Children born to mothers with hepatitis B are at risk of developing the condition themselves.

Causes

As mentioned, hepatitis B is spread through bodily fluids. Therefore, there can be a number of causes of contracting this virus. These include:

- Being born to an infected mother.

- Being in contact with blood or other fluids (e.g., by working in the health care field).

- Being injured or injected by an infected needle (e.g., by using drugs or getting a tattoo).

- Having unprotected sex with an infected individual.

- Sharing a toothbrush, razor, or nail clippers with an infected person.

See a doctor if you suspect you have come into contact with the blood or bodily fluids of an infected person.

Possible Complications

If hepatitis B becomes chronic (lasting longer than six months), serious complications may occur. These complications include developing cirrhosis; an increased risk of liver cancer; and fulminant liver failure.

Diagnosis

The first clues that you may have the condition are elevated liver function tests, as well as a history of contact with either contaminated blood or bodily fluids. If your doctor suspects that you may have hepatitis B, there are tests she may order that are specific to this condition. These tests not only can confirm a hepatitis B diagnosis, but can also establish whether a patient is actively infected or not. Let's review these specialized tests:

Hepatitis B E-antigen

If this test is positive, not only are you acutely infected with this virus, you have the ability to pass the disease onto others. In other words, you are highly infectious.

Hepatitis B E-antibody

If this antibody is positive, your risk of infecting someone else with this virus is very low. You still have active hepatitis B if this antibody is positive, but you are less infectious than you would be if the hepatitis B e-antigen (see page 36) were positive. The hepatitis B e-antibody usually appears after the e-antigen disappears.

Hepatitis B Core Antibody

You are no longer actively infected, but you are on the way to developing permanent antibodies. The development of these antibodies protects you from future infection.

Hepatitis B Surface Antigen

If this is positive, you are still in the acute phase of the virus. If your e-antigen (described on page 36) is negative, however, your risk of infecting others is very low.

Hepatitis B Surface Antibody

This is a test that a doctor will often order after you have been given the hepatitis vaccination series to ensure that you have developed adequate antibodies to this virus.

The time course to the development of the various antibodies is very important. For example, if a person remains hepatitis B e-antigen positive for several months, this implies that the patient is not only at risk of infecting others, but it is likely that the individual also has a high "viral load." This refers to an amount of virus that can be counted, usually in millions of copies. Sustained high viral loads increase the risk of developing chronic hepatitis. Hepatitis B is a DNA virus, so the viral load will measure the amount of hepatitis B in the blood.

Hepatitis B DNA Viral Load

This test measures the viral load of hepatitis B (see section above).

In addition to these tests, doctors can also test the blood to determine which subtype, or genotype, of hepatitis B a patient has (see inset "The Different Genotypes of Hepatitis B" on page 38).

Treatment

If the hepatitis B is acute, the treatment is often conservative and includes getting plenty of rest and drinking water. However, there are times when medical treatment is needed. This happens when there is a persistent elevation of the liver enzymes or if the patient develops acute liver failure due to hepatitis B. Standard therapies include the use of a medication called *interferon*, as well as the use of specialized medications (such as the "nucleoside analogues," discussed below).

There are two types of interferon that are used: *pegylated interferon* and *alpha interferon*. Interferon is a substance that raises the immune system level by activating protective cells that help reduce the viral load. It is given as an injection once weekly under the skin. Side effects can include flu-like symptoms and depression. Because of this, your health care provider may have you screened for depression before prescribing interferon. If you have a history of depression or display any signs that suggest depression, most clinicians will see this as a contraindication (a reason to withhold a certain treatment) to using interferon. If you are felt to be a candidate for interferon treatment but exhibit signs of depression, a consultation with a psychiatric professional may be considered.

Other medications that may be used in the treatment of hepatitis B include *nucleoside analogues*. Examples of these medications include *lamivudine* and *adefovir*. In one study, the use of lamivudine in individuals with cirrhosis due to hepatitis B dramatically reduced the worsening of liver disease. The medication also decreased the risk of developing hepatocel-

The Different Genotypes of Hepatitis B

It is possible to classify further subtypes of hepatitis B. Physicians can send for specialized blood testing to see what type or genotype of hepatitis B is afflicting a patient. There are at least ten different genotypes (genotypes A through J), and these genotypes tend to be region-specific. For example, in Asian countries, genotypes B and C are the most predominant. Studies are undergoing to determine how the understanding of which genotype a patient has can help determine not only what someone's risk may be of developing cirrhosis, but also how well someone may respond to therapy. For example, someone with genotype B may have a lower risk of developing cirrhosis, decreased risk of developing liver cancer, and a better response to treatment (including interferon) than somebody with a different genotype. The combination of genotype identification and the reaction of viral DNA load to treatment can be used to determine if a response to therapy is successful or not.

lular carcinoma (a form of liver cancer). It is important to note that it may take a few months before any improvement in liver function can be seen.

One of the biggest concerns with lamivudine is that resistance to it may develop over time. On page 37, you read about the importance of monitoring viral DNA levels in patients with hepatitis B. One important sign that resistance to lamivudine may be developing is that the viral DNA load begins to increase, despite a patient being on the medication for several months to a year. If this occurs, then the treatment plan will likely need to be modified. Note that lamivudine can be used as the sole therapy for treating hepatitis B, or it can be used in combination with interferon (namely the pegylated interferon).

Adefovir is a pill that can also be used for the treatment of hepatitis B; however, a major side effect of this medication is that it can worsen kidney function.

Like hepatitis A, you can get a vaccination against hepatitis B that provides antibodies and confers protection against this virus. It is a series of three injections given across six months. It is a required vaccination for all health care workers.

Prognosis

Similarly to hepatitis A, the majority of those infected with hepatitis B recover within six months and subsequently become resistant to future exposure to the virus..

However, chronic hepatitis B is associated with not only an increased risk of cirrhosis, but also an increased risk of liver cancer. Children and infants are at higher risk than adults of developing chronic hepatitis B, as they are less able to clear the acute virus. This increases their risk of developing the aforementioned complications.

HEPATITIS C

Hepatitis C is the most common form of viral hepatitis in the United States. Similarly to hepatitis B, it is spread through the bodily fluids of infected patients. It is likely to become chronic.

Signs & Symptoms

In many cases, those who have hepatitis C display no obvious symptoms. An infected person may not know she has the disease for months or even years. However, if hepatitis C develops into cirrhosis, liver cancer, or liver failure, the patient may start feeling sick. Symptoms of hepatitis C include:

- Abdominal swelling (ascites)
- Dark urine
- Fatigue
- Fever
- Jaundice
- Loss of appetite
- Nausea
- Pale stool
- Vomiting

Risk Factors

The risk factors for hepatitis C are similar to those of hepatitis B; both are spread through the exchange of bodily fluids. The people most at risk of contracting hepatitis C include those who share needles that exchange bodily fluids (especially drug users); those who work in the health care field; and babies born to mothers who have the condition.

The risk is also increased for those who have received organ or blood donations, especially before 1992; although blood banks have screened for exposure to the hepatitis C virus since 1992, these tests by themselves are unable to determine if the donor has actually contracted the disease.

Unlike hepatitis B, those who share personal items (such as toothbrushes, razors, or nail clippers) with a person infected with hepatitis C are not at high risk of contracting hepatitis C themselves.

Causes

As mentioned, hepatitis C is spread through bodily fluids. Therefore, there can be a number of causes for contracting this virus. These include:

- Being born to an infected mother.
- Being in contact with blood or other fluids (e.g., by working in the health care field).
- Being injured or injected by an infected needle (e.g., by using drugs or getting a tattoo).
- Having unprotected sex with an infected individual.
- Sharing a toothbrush, razor, or nail clippers with an infected person (uncommon).

See a doctor if you suspect you have come into contact with the blood or bodily fluids of an infected person. Additionally, if you were born between 1945 and 1965, your doctor will likely discuss your undergoing testing for hepatitis C. According to the Centers for Disease Control and Prevention (CDC), people born in this time period are five times more likely than others to be infected with this virus.

Possible Complications

Hepatitis C is a medical condition that has the potential to affect other organs in the body. The complications do not occur in everyone, but it is important to recognize them. The other conditions associated with hepatitis C can include:

Cryoglobulinemia

Cryoglobulinemia (*cry-o-glob-you-lin-nee-mia*) is an inflammation of the blood vessels that can also cause a skin rash, usually in the lower extremities. It occurs when abnormal proteins clump together and build up in the blood, restricting blood flow.

Kidney Disease

Hepatitis C can cause an inflammatory reaction in the kidneys called *nephritis* (*neh-fry-tis*) in a small percentage of individuals. The kidney disease associated with hepatitis C often occurs with cryoglobulinemia (see above). The abnormal proteins associated with cryoglobulinemia are the antibody type of proteins, which contribute to the intense inflammatory reaction in the kidney.

Skin Conditions

There can be several skin conditions associated with hepatitis C. One of the most common is cryoglobulinemia (above). There can be skin lesions called *purpura* on the legs. These skin lesions are caused by inflamed blood vessels.

Vasculitis

This is an inflammation of the blood vessels. Cryoglobulinemia is an example of a serious vasculitis that is associated with hepatitis C.

Diagnosis

In addition to taking a patient history to assess any risk factors, there are many tests used to diagnose hepatitis C. These include antibody tests, RNA tests, and possibly a biopsy. One of the first indications that you may have hepatitis C is an elevation in the liver function tests, especially the ALT (alanine aminotransferase) level.

Usually, a doctor will confirm hepatitis C by ordering a test for the antibodies that fight against hepatitis C. Note that if you have risk factors but the initial test for antibodies comes back negative, your doctor may re-test you on a later date, as you may have the condition but not yet have formed antibodies. Antibodies can take two to three months to form after the virus first enters the body. The antibody test can tell your doctor whether your body has cleared the hepatitis C virus. If the antibody test is negative, but your doctor still suspects a hepatitis C diagnosis, a viral load test may be ordered.

The viral load test, also called the HCV RNA test, can confirm a hepatitis C diagnosis. The test examines your bloodstream for the virus. The quantitative version of the test can also determine how much of the virus is in your blood. A higher viral load suggests a higher resistance to treatment. The viral load test is helpful in determining what kind of treatment should be used and for how long. The test can be performed again some time after treatment is given to evaluate the treatment's effectiveness.

The blood can also be tested for high levels of bilirubin, liver enzymes, and the proteins of the liver function test that you read about in Chapter 2 (including alanine and alkaline phosphatase). However, these tests are not specific to hepatitis C, and further testing may still be needed if these levels are found to be unusual.

Occasionally, a liver biopsy may be taken. This is normally done after a hepatitis C diagnosis is confirmed; the biopsy determines how damaged the liver may be.

Treatment

Not everyone who is diagnosed with hepatitis C needs treatment. For example, if the tests for ALT (alanine aminotransferase) are normal, and there is a minimal viral load on the RNA test, then you may not require treatment. Meanwhile, if you have an elevation in your liver tests and/or have an elevated viral load, your doctor may recommend treatment. Sometimes your doctor will order a liver biopsy to determine the amount of liver inflammation and fibrosis in the liver. Note that while obtaining a liver biopsy is not unusual, it is also not a standard practice. Recall from Chapter 2 that a newer type of ultrasound test, called ultrasound elastography, can be performed to help determine the presence and severity of liver fibrosis (scarring). Many doctors will elect to discuss different treatment options with you given the presence of a significant viral load.

Understanding which genotype of hepatitis C you have is very important because it can help determine how well you will respond to treatment. Unlike hepatitis B, where the different genotypes are named after letters (see "The Different Genotypes of Hepatitis B" inset on page 38), the genotypes of hepatitis C are classified using a numerical system. The genotypes range from 1 to 6. This is not a "severity score" (i.e., type 1 is not the least severe and type 6 is not the most severe). Rather, they represent different "types" of hepatitis C.

In the United States, for example, 1 is the most common genotype identified. That being said, if someone with this hepatitis C has this genotype, they may not respond as readily to treatment as someone with types 2 or 3 (these types are more receptive to treatment).

Treatment options include the use of three medications: interferon, *ribavirin (rye-buh-vye-rin)*, and a class of medications called *serine protease inhibitors.* All three of them can be used together for the treatment of hepatitis C. Usually, these medications are prescribed for an average of six to nine months. The form of interferon used is pegylated interferon (see page 38). It is often prescribed as a once-weekly injection.

Ribavirin is an antiviral medication. Because this medication can cause suppression of your bone marrow, causing anemia, low platelets, and low white cell counts, your blood cell counts will be monitored closely if you are taking this medication.

Serine protease inhibitors are a relatively new class of medications prescribed for hepatitis C. They act by not only inhibiting the replication of the hepatitis C virus (to help reduce the viral load), but they also enable the interferon to be more potent than it would be without this additional medication. Examples of this new class of medications include telaprevir (brand names Incivek and Incivo) and sofosbuvir (brand name Sovaldi).

Prognosis

This is a very common form of both acute and chronic hepatitis. Hepatitis C becomes chronic in about 75 to 85 percent of cases, according to the CDC.

In addition to obtaining follow-up blood work to further evaluate the viral load, it is recommended that an ultrasound of the liver and a special lab test called an *alpha-fetoprotein level* be obtained every six months. This is because hepatitis C can increase the risk of developing hepatocellular carcinoma. The lab test plus the ultrasound is part of the screening for this condition.

To further protect the liver, it is recommended you get vaccinated against hepatitis A and B (see inset "The Need for Hepatitis Immunizations" on page 45).

OTHER CAUSES OF VIRAL HEPATITIS

Hepatitis A, B, and C are the most common causes of viral hepatitis, but there are additional viruses that can cause this condition. These include the less common forms of hepatitis (types D and E) and Epstein-Barr virus (EBV).

Hepatitis D

Hepatitis D only occurs in individuals who already have hepatitis B (see page 35). About 15 to 20 million people who have hepatitis B also develop hepatitis D. Having both hepatitis B and D can weaken the liver and cause a more dangerous and chronic liver disease, such as cirrhosis.

Treatment options can include pegylated interferon (see page 38). Some studies suggest that the combination of interferon and adefovir (see page 39) may be beneficial; the studies are ongoing. Liver transplant (see Chapter 7) is an option if acute fulminant liver failure, liver cancer, or advanced cirrhosis develops. The strongest defense against contracting the hepatitis D virus is to get the hepatitis B vaccine, which protects the patient from both infections.

Hepatitis E

Hepatitis E is transmitted through contaminated water, similar to hepatitis A. Coming into contact with domestic pigs is another common source of hepatitis E. Person-to-person transmission (other than from mother to child in birth) is rare. Organ transplant recipients whose immune systems have been compromised (usually due to medication that prevents organ rejection) are considered the highest group at risk of contracting hepatitis E. Hepatitis E is more common in developing countries. Vaccines are in the process of being developed and tested. In the majority of cases, hep-

The Need for Hepatitis Immunizations

If you have hepatitis C, it is important to be immunized against hepatitis A and hepatitis B. The hepatitis A vaccination usually consists of two doses (the first after the age of one, the second at least six months later). The hepatitis B vaccination is a series of three injections given over a period of a few months. The importance of vaccinations that prevent you from acquiring other forms of hepatitis if you have hepatitis C cannot be emphasized enough. Again, you want to do all that you can to protect your liver.

atitis E is acute and goes away on its own. However, between 1 and 4 percent of hepatitis E cases become fatal; this statistic can jump to 25 percent in pregnant women.

Epstein-Barr Virus (EBV)

Epstein-Barr virus (EBV) is one of the most common viruses in the world. It can affect as many as 90 percent of adults worldwide, although it often causes no symptoms. However, in a small percentage of cases, it can cause acute hepatitis. While this is uncommon, physicians will evaluate a patient for EBV if the more common causes of viral hepatitis have been ruled out. Patients who have hepatitis caused by EBV can present with the symptoms already mentioned in Chapter 2, including jaundice and an enlarged liver.

EBV is transferred through saliva and once infected, most people develop immunity to it (although the virus remains latent in the cells). When it does become active, it is responsible for the onset of many illnesses, including mononucleosis ("mono"). This is very common in school-aged men and women. Mono is characterized by the presence of a sore throat (*pharyngitis*) with accompanying "white stuff" (*exudates*) that your doctor can see when she looks at your tonsils. It also can cause fatigue, malaise, and joint and body aches. On examination, doctors often find the presence of a large spleen.

The treatment for EBV is supportive; affected individuals are often advised to refrain from contact sports or engaging in serious physical exercise for at least six weeks, which is about how long it can take to recover from mono. Unfortunately, there is no prescription medication that can be given for either mononucleosis or EBV-induced hepatitis.

ALCOHOLIC HEPATITIS

In the previous section, I discussed viral hepatitis and the viruses that cause it—hepatitis A, B, C, D, and E, as well as Epstein-Barr virus. There is also a form of hepatitis that is not caused by a virus, called *alcoholic hepatitis*. As the name implies, this condition is caused by excessive drinking.

SIGNS AND SYMPTOMS

As in viral hepatitis, alcoholic hepatitis causes inflammation and swelling of the liver. Alcoholic hepatitis shares many symptoms with the viral type. These include:

- Abdominal tenderness
- Fever (often mild)
- Generalized fatigue
- Jaundice
- Loss of appetite
- Nausea/vomiting
- Weakness
- Weight loss

Severe alcoholic hepatitis may show these additional symptoms:

- Ascites (fluid buildup in the abdomen)
- Confusion or other behavioral changes
- Kidney and/or liver failure

Additionally, the majority of those with alcoholic hepatitis suffer from malnutrition (because alcohol suppresses their appetite and is their main source of calories) and toxin buildup (which prevents absorption of nutrients).

RISK FACTORS

Heavy alcohol consumption is the main risk factor for alcoholic hepatitis. Most who develop the condition have a history of drinking the equivalent of seven drinks a day, every day.

Other risk factors include gender (alcohol is processed differently in women, and so women have a higher risk of developing alcoholic hepatitis); weight (being overweight or obese increases the chance of developing alcoholic hepatitis); and binge drinking (consuming five or more drinks in one day, even if it is not a daily occurrence). Genetics and race can also play a role in developing alcoholic hepatitis, although it is difficult to separate biological and environmental factors.

CAUSES

Alcoholic hepatitis is caused by excessive alcohol consumption that damages the liver. When the liver breaks down alcohol, toxic chemicals are produced. One such chemical is *acetaldehyde*, which can be toxic in large amounts. Chemicals such as acetaldehyde cause inflammation and damage to the liver cells.

POSSIBLE COMPLICATIONS

Alcoholic hepatitis can cause a number of complications in the rest of the body, including:

- Ascites.

- Cognitive damage, such as confusion and slurred speech, due to a buildup of toxins that the liver is unable to remove.

- Enlarged veins, which occur when blood that cannot easily flow into the liver backs up into other, thinner blood vessels. If these blood vessels burst, it causes internal bleeding in the stomach or esophagus, which is life-threatening.

- High blood pressure in the liver, or portal hypertension (due to inflammation and scarring that slows down blood flow in the liver).

- Kidney failure.

DIAGNOSIS

Many of the tests mentioned in Chapter 2 can be used to diagnose alcoholic hepatitis. These include a physical examination (looking for an enlarged liver), liver function tests, blood tests, an ultrasound, a CT scan, an MRI scan, or a liver biopsy. An accurate, honest patient history that describes the patient's drinking habits is important in diagnosing alcoholic hepatitis (see "The CAGE Questionnaire for Alcoholism" inset on page 48). The Maddrey discriminant function (MDF) is often used by clinicians to determine the severity of the alcoholic hepatitis and the type of therapy that is needed (see page 49).

The CAGE Questionnaire for Alcoholism

There are various questionnaires that health care professionals will employ to try and find out if someone has a drinking problem. One of the most common techniques is the CAGE questionnaire. Each letter of the acronym stands for a different question:

C Are you or others concerned about your drinking habits?

A Do you get angry or annoyed when people talk to you about your drinking habits?

G Do you ever feel guilt or remorse concerning your own drinking habits?

E Do you ever need to have the so-called "eye-opener"— an alcoholic beverage first thing in the morning to prevent the "morning shakes" after a night of drinking?

If the answer is "yes" to two or more questions, this is a strong indication that the patient may have a drinking problem. The CAGE questionnaire has been studied extensively and is felt to be an effective screening tool for the diagnosis of alcohol abuse.

TREATMENT

The only possible way to prevent alcoholic hepatitis from becoming fatal (or even to reverse the liver damage) is to stop drinking alcohol completely. Treatments for the symptoms and complications may be given, but if the patient continues to drink alcohol, these treatments will not be effective and liver damage will continue to worsen.

Those who are dependent on alcohol may be recommended therapies such as counseling, participation in an Alcoholics Anonymous group, or an outpatient program.

The doctor may also give treatments for malnutrition, such as vitamins or tube feeding. Anti-inflammatory medications such as corticosteroids or pentoxifylline (brand name Trental) may be given to treat liver inflammation, although the effectiveness and safety of these medications are not clear.

In severe, fatal cases, a liver transplant may be performed to prevent death. However, it is difficult to obtain a liver transplant, especially for alcoholics. This is because the centers that perform liver transplants are fearful that the patient will resume drinking after surgery. Many centers have requirements that must be met (e.g., not drinking alcohol for at least six months before the surgery) before transplantation is considered.

PROGNOSIS

Alcoholic hepatitis is a very severe disease. It is important to realize that acute alcoholic hepatitis can be associated with increased morbidity and mortality. The thirty-day mortality rate of those who have advanced alcoholic hepatitis is estimated to be 30 to 40 percent. Mortality is accelerated by continued drinking—even if it is just "one drink a day" (see inset below).

There are various scoring systems that physicians will use to help determine the severity of the alcoholic hepatitis at the time of presentation. The most commonly used system is the Maddrey discriminant function (MDF), mentioned on page 47. This is a formula clinicians use to get an idea of the severity of the alcoholic hepatitis. If the score on the MDF is greater than 32, the patient's risk of mortality increases by one-third; she is also considered to be a candidate for treatment, such as steroids.

Over time, alcoholic hepatitis can cause scarring of the liver tissue, also known as cirrhosis (see page 54). Cirrhosis is a chronic, irreversible condition, and is especially damaging when it is alcohol-induced.

It can be very difficult to stop drinking. If you find yourself or a loved one in this situation, some excellent sources for help can be found on page 185 in the Resources section.

The "One a Day" Misconception

Many books and health care providers claim that a small amount of alcohol—a glass of red wine a day, for example—is "healthy." The thought behind this, as far as red wine is concerned, is that a primary ingredient called *resveratrol* provides health benefits that could be obtained by consuming red wine. This statement has been reconsidered because of the risk to the liver of consuming alcohol daily. If you want the benefits of red wine, taking a resveratrol supplement may be your best option. From a health perspective, it is no longer recommended to have that "daily cocktail"—especially if you are at risk for or exhibit signs of liver disease.

NON-ALCOHOLIC FATTY LIVER DISEASE
AND NON-ALCOHOLIC STEATOHEPATITIS

Fatty liver has recently surpassed excessive alcohol consumption as the most common cause of liver disease. Fatty liver is just what its name says: It is the accumulation of fat in the cells of the liver. The fat cells are called *adipocytes* (*add-dip-o-sites*) and the liver cells are called *hepatocytes* (*hep-ah-toe-sites*). Fat accumulation in the liver cells is a process that can take months to years. A liver is considered to be a fatty liver if more than 5 to 10 percent of its weight is fat.

There are two forms of this condition that we will discuss in this section. The first is *non-alcoholic fatty liver disease* (NAFLD). A person with NAFLD can have a fatty liver without any signs of inflammation or hepatitis. In other words, a patient with NAFLD will have normal blood tests when her liver function is assessed. The increase in obesity rates, as well as the epidemic number of individuals with diabetes, have significantly contributed to the rise of NAFLD.

The other form of this condition is called *non-alcoholic steatohepatitis* (*stee-at-toe hepatitis*), or NASH. This is when fatty liver transitions into hepatitis. NASH is a severe subset of NAFLD. The initial sign of an acute hepatitis is that there is an elevation in the blood work, especially the alanine transasminase (ALT) and aspartate transaminase (AST) levels. Ultrasound imaging of the liver can also suggest that a person has a fatty liver, as "fat lobules" can be seen on the ultrasound. The ultrasound findings will be similar in both NAFLD and NASH. Refer back to Chapter 2 for more detailed explanations of the blood work and imaging studies that are used to evaluate the liver.

One study from the journal *Gastroenterology* estimated the prevalence of non-alcoholic fatty liver disease to be about 46 percent and non-alcoholic steatohepatitis to be about 14 to 18 percent. This was a study that enrolled 328 people with an age range of twenty-eight to seventy. All of the study participants filled out a questionnaire and underwent a liver ultrasound. If there was evidence of a fatty liver on the ultrasound, then further blood testing and a biopsy of the liver were performed to confirm the presence of fatty liver disease in those subjects.

SIGNS AND SYMPTOMS

NAFLD and NASH typically do not exhibit signs or symptoms. Fatigue, abdominal pain, weakness, and weight loss may be experienced occasionally.

RISK FACTORS

Risk factors for the development of a fatty liver or NASH include:

- Chronic alcohol use (while alcohol is a direct risk factor for alcohol-related liver disease, its consumption can also increase the risk of developing a fatty liver).

- High blood pressure

- High cholesterol levels

- High triglyceride levels

- Leaky gut (permeable intestines)

- Metabolic syndrome (simultaneous onset of increased blood pressure, high blood sugar, excess body fat in the waist area, and excessively high or low cholesterol levels)

- Obesity

- Pre-existing diabetes

- Poor diet

Genetics may play a role as well. In the *Gastroenterology* study mentioned on page 50, approximately 60 percent of the subjects who were of Hispanic ethnicity were found to have fatty liver disease. The next most affected group was Caucasians, then African-Americans. One of the most significant findings from that study was that of those patients who had been diagnosed with diabetes, approximately 75 percent were diagnosed with having fatty liver disease as well.

CAUSES

Because NAFLD and NASH are prevalent in a number of diseases and can be the result of a number of different factors, it is difficult to pinpoint an exact cause for either. They are primarily linked to poor diet, obesity, and diabetes; insulin resistance is also thought to be related. Secondary causes can include malnutrition; certain medications (e.g., antivirals and corticosteroids); metabolic disorders; toxins; and infections, such as hepatitis C.

POSSIBLE COMPLICATIONS

NAFLD and NASH typically do not cause complications. However, it is important to note that in the most severe cases of NAFLD and especially NASH, cirrhosis or liver cancer can develop.

DIAGNOSIS

As NAFLD and NASH do not typically present symptoms, diagnosis is most often made through testing. These include liver function tests and imaging procedures such as an ultrasound, CT scan, or MRI scan. A liver biopsy is the best way to determine whether the patient has NAFLD and whether it has progressed to NASH, as well as the extent of fibrosis (scarring) that may be present.

Several studies have examined the prognostic importance of uric acid in the setting of fatty liver disease. A 2014 study from the journal *Clinical Biochemistry* examined approximately 240 patients diagnosed with fatty liver disease, ranging from a benign fatty liver to the development of NASH. The authors found that one-third of the patients had high uric acid levels. Those with NASH had higher uric acid levels than those with a benign fatty liver. Other factors associated with a higher uric acid level included obesity and age (being younger was associated with high uric acid levels).

If you have elevated uric acid levels and other risk factors associated with the development of a fatty liver, then you and your doctor should discuss having an ultrasound and further evaluation of your liver performed (see "Fatty Liver: Redefining Preventative Care" inset on page 53).

TREATMENT

The treatment for a fatty liver first requires the diagnosis of the underlying cause. If metabolic syndrome (high blood pressure, high blood sugar,

Fatty Liver: Redefining Preventative Care

When it comes to causes of liver disease, NAFLD and NASH are likely more predominant than we are aware of. If we were to expand the results of the prevalence study mentioned on page 50 to the general population, over 75 percent of people diagnosed with diabetes would also have NAFLD. Of those, 25 percent would have NASH.

In most cases, a fatty liver is diagnosed only after an elevation of the liver enzymes is found and when acute inflammation and hepatitis are already present. However, the issue with this is that a fatty liver can persist for a long time before acute hepatitis develops (if it develops at all). If an ultrasound of the liver is ordered by a physician, it is often for another reason. For example, if a doctor suspects that a gallbladder disease may be present in a patient who actually has NAFLD, the fatty liver is then found incidentally because of the liver's close proximity to the gallbladder.

If someone has risk factors for the development of a fatty liver—especially if she already has diabetes—it is my personal belief that an ultrasound of the liver should be ordered, even in the setting of normal liver function tests. If this condition is detected early, then (with the appropriate nutritional and lifestyle interventions) its onset can perhaps be delayed or even averted. While this is not yet the recommended standard of preventative care concerning NAFLD and NASH, I believe it should be.

and excessively high or low cholesterol levels), obesity, and/or diabetes are present, a significant lifestyle change is recommended. This includes implementing healthy eating habits and engaging in a daily exercise plan. Detailed dietary suggestions and exercise plans are covered in Part Two of this book. Start small—rapid weight loss can be just as harmful as weight gain to NAFLD and NASH. Natural supplements (described in Chapter 10) may help liver function, although you should consult with a doctor first; some supplements may interfere with prescribed medication. As with all liver diseases, avoid alcohol consumption.

PROGNOSIS

Prognosis of NAFLD and NASH depends on the severity of the disease. A fatty liver on its own is relatively benign, but if steatohepatitis is present, the chance of developing worsening liver disease increases. In particular, steatohepatitis can lead to cirrhosis, which is irreversible and leads to long-term damage.

CIRRHOSIS

As discussed in Chapter 2, cirrhosis is an ongoing and irreversible condition that can be fatal. Its signature symptom is the scarring of the liver cells. This scarring is due to chronic damage; each time the liver experiences damage, it tries to repair itself. Scar tissue forms in the process. The scarring affects the liver's blood flow and pressure systems. If the liver's circulation and pressure are affected, it can negatively affect the rest of the body's ability to fight even a mild sickness.

SIGNS AND SYMPTOMS

The symptoms of cirrhosis are similar to the symptoms of many of the other liver diseases we have discussed in this chapter. The symptoms may not be present in the early stages of cirrhosis, but may become more pronounced as the condition progresses:

- Ascites (fluid buildup in the abdomen, leading to a "pregnant" appearance)
- Edema (fluid buildup in the legs or ankles)
- Fatigue and weakness
- Itching
- Jaundice
- Loss of appetite
- Nausea
- Spider angiomas (spider-like blood vessels visible on the skin)
- Weight loss

If you have these symptoms, particularly ascites and edema, and suspect you may have cirrhosis, see a doctor right away.

RISK FACTORS

Risk factors for cirrhosis include:

- Age (cirrhosis is more common in those over 50 years of age)
- Frequent alcohol consumption

- Having pre-existing hepatitis (especially types B and C) or fatty liver

- Genetic factors, such as hemochromatosis or Wilson's disease (see page 66)

- Gender (a higher number of males than females develop cirrhosis)

- Obesity

CAUSES

Cirrhosis is most commonly caused by the progression of another liver disease. Hepatitis C, alcohol abuse, and fatty liver are the most common causes of cirrhosis. As you may recall, hepatitis C is transmitted through exposure to contaminated blood and often becomes chronic. It may not display any symptoms until it becomes more severe; people may not realize they have hepatitis C until after cirrhosis has been diagnosed.

Hepatitis B, which is also spread through contaminated blood, is a common cause of cirrhosis worldwide. However, in the United States, it is much less common (affecting less than one percent of the population). As with hepatitis C, many people do not realize they have hepatitis B until they find out that it has caused cirrhosis.

Alcoholism is second only to chronic hepatitis C as the most common cause of cirrhosis in the United States. The amount of alcohol that is generally thought to cause cirrhosis is more than two drinks a day (women) or three drinks a day (men) daily for ten to twelve years. Even if the liver has been afflicted with a non-alcohol-related condition (such as acute viral hepatitis), alcohol consumption of any kind can cause further damage to the liver and prevent it from healing itself.

Non-alcoholic steatohepatitis (NASH), discussed in the section beginning on page 50, is the third most common cause of cirrhosis in the United States. It is the severe subset of non-alcoholic fatty liver disease (NAFLD). NASH leads to inflammation (and therefore, scarring) of the liver, which is why it is more likely to cause cirrhosis than NAFLD.

There are other, less common causes of cirrhosis, including biliary diseases and conditions. These include *primary biliary cirrhosis, primary sclerosing cholangitis,* and gallstones; each causes damage to the ducts that bring bile out of the liver and into the small intestine. When the biliary ducts are inflamed, hardened, blocked, or otherwise injured, bile backs up into the liver and causes cirrhosis.

Genetic diseases, namely hemochromatosis and Wilson's disease, can negatively affect how the liver processes proteins, minerals, and other substances. Buildup of these substances can cause cirrhosis. (See "Hemochromatosis" and "Wilson's Disease" on pages 66 and 68 for more details on these conditions.)

Up to 20 percent of cirrhosis cases are deemed *cryptogenic cirrhosis* (*crip-toe-genic*). When someone is diagnosed with cryptogenic cirrhosis, it means that the doctor cannot find the cause behind the cirrhosis.

POSSIBLE COMPLICATIONS

Because cirrhosis alters the liver's blood flow and pressure systems, there are many possible complications that can affect other important organs in the body. Sometimes, the complications are actually the first indicator that somebody has cirrhosis.

In Chapter 2, I briefly discussed portal hypertension. This is a possible complication in which the liver's scar tissue blocks blood flow and increases the pressure in the portal vein. The portal vein delivers blood to the liver from the spleen and intestines, providing about 75 percent of the liver's nutrients. The increase in pressure leads to the telltale signs of liver disease: ascites and edema. Ascites, in turn, can cause *bacterial peritonitis*, a serious infection that affects the fluid in the abdomen.

When pressure in the portal vein increases, the spleen may become enlarged as well. This is called *splenomegaly*. If the spleen is enlarged, it can hoard excess white blood cells and platelets (blood clotting cells) and keep them from being released into the patient's bloodstream. This is why a blood test can help diagnose cirrhosis; if the blood test shows a low white blood cell count or a low platelet count, it is a signal that something may be wrong with the liver.

Portal hypertension can also cause *varices*—enlarged blood vessels—in the esophagus and stomach. When pressure increases in the portal vein, blood flow is redirected to smaller vessels. Because these veins are taking on more blood flow than their size allows, their walls become thin; they can burst and cause internal bleeding if the pressure becomes too high. This is a serious complication that requires medical attention, especially if the liver's ability to clot blood has been compromised.

Another severe complication of cirrhosis is *hepatic encephalopathy (en-seff-uh-lop-uh-thee)*. This is a condition in which the liver cannot properly remove toxins from the bloodstream; the toxins then build up in the brain. Toxin buildup can cause decreased mental function; confusion; changes in personality and/or sleeping habits; memory loss; trouble focusing; and, in rare cases, coma.

Other possible complications of cirrhosis include: malnutrition (because the liver is unable to properly process nutrients); bone diseases and loss of bone strength (due to lack of nutrients, such as calcium and vitamin D); bruising and bleeding; gallstones; liver cancer; and multi-organ failure.

DIAGNOSIS

As early-stage cirrhosis often does not show any symptoms, a doctor may order tests for cirrhosis based on existing risk factors (such as obesity, diabetes, or alcoholism). A patient history is usually the first thing a doctor will consider for diagnosis. The patient history can detail a patient's drinking, eating, or smoking habits, as well as any inherited conditions that could cause cirrhosis.

Next, the doctor may perform a physical examination to check for a liver that feels hardened. The doctor will also look for signs of swelling in the abdomen or legs due to excess fluid (ascites and edema).

Blood tests, imaging tests, and a biopsy can be used to confirm a diagnosis of cirrhosis. As you may recall from Chapter 2, the blood tests looks for unusual levels of liver enzymes, bilirubin, creatinine (which is a sign of impaired kidney function), and blood clotting factors. The blood tests can be used to calculate how much time a patient with end-stage liver disease will have to live.

Imaging tests include the ultrasound, CT scan, or MRI scan. These tests use different methods to produce detailed images of the liver. The images show the doctor any abnormalities in the liver surface. An ultrasound can best show the development of cirrhosis over time, including the presence of a small, shrunken liver.

Elastography, a test that is fairly new and is gaining popularity, is a non-invasive way to measure the stiffness of the liver (livers with more scar tissue are more stiff). This is done using an ultrasound or an MRI scan. Studies are ongoing to determine its ability to detect and evaluate the degree of fibrosis in liver disease. The results are encouraging in the use of ultrasound to help evaluate for the possibility of fibrosis, especially in patients with viral hepatitis.

A biopsy is perhaps the most accurate indicator, not only of a diagnosis, but also the severity and extent of the condition. The biopsy involves removing a small piece of tissue from the liver via a needle. An alternative procedure to a biopsy, called a Fibroscan, is a non-invasive study that can help determine if cirrhosis is present or not. In one study, the results of this scan were compared to biopsy results in patients with viral hepatitis. The results demonstrated that the Fibroscan can reliably measure the extent of fibrosis in the liver.

TREATMENT

While the scarring in the liver cells is irreversible, steps can be taken to prevent further damage and complications. Treating the underlying cause of the cirrhosis is vital. Alcohol must be avoided completely. It is important to follow a healthy diet because of the risks of malnutrition and malabsorption of vitamins and minerals.

If hepatitis is the underlying cause (and even if it is not), the patient should be given a vaccination. Vaccines are available for types A and B. Although there is no vaccine for hepatitis C, patients who are at risk for liver disease can get blood screening tests for early detection. Antiviral medication can be taken to treat hepatitis B or C.

All medication and supplements, even over-the-counter drugs, should be taken under the supervision of a doctor. Cirrhosis decreases the liver's ability to filter medication from the blood. The medication then can build up in the body, causing more damage to the liver.

In many cases, medications are given to treat the complications and symptoms of cirrhosis. These include beta blockers or nitrates for portal hypertension and varices; diuretics for ascites and edema (diuretics reduce the amount of fluid in the body); antibiotics for bacterial peritonitis; and laxatives for hepatic encephalopathy. (I will go into more detail about these medications in Chapter 5.) Nutritional supplements or vitamins may be recommended to make up for the liver's inability to provide nutrients to the rest of the body. These should also be taken under the supervision of a doctor; it is possible to "overdose" on certain vitamins.

If cirrhosis progresses into liver cancer, treatment for cancer may be given. Treatment can include surgery, radiation therapy, or chemotherapy. A patient with liver disease should be screened once or twice a year for signs of liver cancer. (See section "Liver Cancer" on page 59 for more information on this topic.)

Surgical procedures may be necessary in some cases. If gallstones emerge as a complication, surgery can be done to remove them or to remove the gallbladder entirely. Surgery can also be performed to redirect blood flow and prevent portal hypertension. In the most severe cases of cirrhosis (e.g., if liver failure is imminent), a liver transplant may be required. This is the best treatment, as the liver being transplanted into the patient will have no scarring, but it is difficult to obtain.

PROGNOSIS

Cirrhosis is a chronic (lasting longer than six months), ongoing condition. Prognosis depends on the underlying cause. For example, if cirrhosis is caused by alcoholism, the chances of recovery increase once the patient stops drinking completely. If hepatitis C is the cause, antiviral medications can slow the damage.

A scoring system called the *Child-Pugh score* can be used to determine the prognosis of the cirrhosis. The Child-Pugh system measures (on a scale of 1 to 3) the severity of five categories (total bilirubin, serum albumin, prothrombin time, ascites, and hepatic encephalopathy). The points are added up to determine if the cirrhosis falls into Child-Pugh class A, B, or C. Class A has the highest rate of survival after two years, while class C has the lowest.

Cirrhosis cannot be completely cured, but if early detection and treatment is undergone, it can prevent the condition from becoming any worse. On the other hand, if complications such as internal bleeding or liver cancer occur, cirrhosis can progress into life-threatening liver failure. A liver transplant is the only way to recover from liver failure.

LIVER CANCER

Liver cancer is one of the most common cancers in the world. Sometimes, the cancer starts in the liver (primary liver cancer). More often, cancer in the liver has been spread there from another part of the body (metastatic liver cancer). There are different types of liver cancer; the most common (occurring in about 75 percent of liver cancer cases) is called *hepatocellular carcinoma*. The details of liver cancer are beyond the scope of this book, but here we will briefly discuss the most important aspects.

SIGNS AND SYMPTOMS

The symptoms of liver cancer are similar to those of other liver diseases. Many of these diseases, such as cirrhosis, can progress into cancer if they are undetected or untreated for too long. This is why it is so important to get screened for the presence of possible hepatocellular carcinoma, especially if you have predisposing conditions (such as hepatitis C). Early detection of liver cancer is key for treatment, so it is vital to go to the doctor as soon as you notice symptoms. These include:

- Abdominal pain, especially on the upper right-hand side

- Ascites

- Bruising

- Enlarged liver (able to be felt under the right-side rib cage)

- Fatigue and generalized weakness

- Feeling full after a small meal

- Itching

- Jaundice

- Loss of appetite

- Nausea or vomiting

- Unexplained weight loss

Cancerous tumors can cause other symptoms, depending on any hormones they may release. These symptoms include:

- High calcium level, which can cause nausea, confusion, and weakness.

- High cholesterol level.

- High red blood cell count or high hemoglobin level (leading to a flushed-looking face).

- Low blood sugar level, which causes fatigue, lethargy, and confusion. (This symptom can occur in advanced cirrhosis as well, as the liver undergoes trouble with glucose production.)

RISK FACTORS

Risk factors for liver disease include:

- **Age.** More than 95 percent of those who have been diagnosed with liver cancer are over forty-five years of age, and only about 2 percent of patients are under age thirty-five.

- **Alcoholism.** As I have discussed, alcohol abuse can severely damage the liver and make it more susceptible to cancer.

- **Existing liver disease.** Some cases of hepatitis, cirrhosis, hemochromatosis, and Wilson's disease progress into liver cancer.

- **Gender.** Males make up about 70 percent of the population who have been diagnosed with liver cancer.

- **Genetics.** Asian Americans and Pacific Islanders have the highest rates of liver cancer in the United States.

CAUSES

Cancer in general is caused when cells become damaged. The cells carry DNA, as well as genes that instruct the cells how often to grow, divide, or when to die off. When these genes become deformed, cells replicate too quickly and become cancerous.

Although there are several risk factors for developing liver cancer, it is unknown what exactly causes it. Exposure to some chemicals called *aflatoxins* can damage liver cells. These chemicals are produced by molds that grow in soil and grains that are stored outdoors.

Hepatitis viruses have their own, viral DNA, which can alter the DNA of the liver cells and tell them to reproduce more often than is necessary.

Cancer sometimes is spread to the liver from another part of the body. For example, cells from breast cancer or lung cancer can spread to the liver. If you have already been diagnosed with another cancer, it is recommended that you talk with your doctor about whether it has spread to your liver.

POSSIBLE COMPLICATIONS

Liver cancer itself can be a complication from another, pre-existing liver disease. However, liver cancer also comes with its own complications. These usually involve tumors, if they are present. When the tumors grow and spread, they can affect other parts of the body. They can also block and back up the flow of bile out of the liver. Other complications include decreased appetite, fever, and weight loss. In the late stages of cancer, liver failure may occur.

Liver cancer may spread to nearby parts of the body, such as the stomach or the lungs. This occurs in late-stage cancer.

Complications can also occur from liver cancer treatments (see "Treatment" below). When surgery is undergone, patients may experience complications from the anesthesia, infection, or internal bleeding. Radiation and chemotherapy are two of the most common cancer treatments, but they are not entirely localized; they may cause damage to healthy cells and lead to liver function deterioration. Additionally, chemotherapy may affect the ovaries and lead to infertility in some women. Chemotherapy often causes hair loss.

DIAGNOSIS

Liver cancer can be difficult to diagnose early because patients often do not experience troubling symptoms until the cancer has entered a late stage. Tumors can go undetected because the liver is covered by the rib cage, which may obscure any abnormalities. If you are at risk for liver cancer—especially if you already have hepatitis, cirrhosis, or another diagnosed liver disease—a screening test once or twice a year is recommended for preventative care.

Screening consists of blood tests and an ultrasound. The blood test looks for a protein called *alpha-fetoprotein,* or AFP. This protein is elevated in the setting of liver cancer. However, many patients with liver cancer have normal AFP levels; AFP can also be elevated in other cancers or noncancerous conditions. Therefore, an ultrasound is recommended to go along with this test. The ultrasound can show any tumors or abnormalities inside the liver.

CT and MRI scans can also be used to take images of the liver. A liver biopsy can be performed if there is a lesion (abnormality or damage) seen in the liver, and your doctor suspects that it may be caused by cancer.

TREATMENT

There are several treatment options that can be used to treat liver cancer. These include surgery to remove the cancer; radiation therapy; embolization; and chemotherapy.

If the cancer is able to be operated on (see "Resectable Stages" on page 65), a surgery called a *partial hepatectomy* can be performed to remove it without requiring a liver transplant. This is a serious surgery that must be performed by an experienced professional. The cancerous part of the liver must be removed, but enough of the liver must be left in for the body to function properly. There is a possibility of the cancer returning after the surgery. This is because cancer is often caused by an underlying condition in the liver that can recur, even after surgery.

If surgery is not possible, *radiation therapy* can be performed. Radiation therapy consists of concentrated, high-energy rays that are used to kill off the cancerous cells. The doctor will determine how much radiation to give, as well as the exact location to which the radiation will be delivered. Radiation treatment only takes a few minutes and is similar to getting an X-ray. However, they are given very often—usually five days a week for several weeks. Radiation also cannot be given at high doses because it can damage healthy liver cells. Technology is emerging to ensure radiation hits the tumors and avoids the normal cells.

A more local treatment is *embolization,* which is the blockage of the hepatic artery to reduce blood flow to the cancerous liver cells. Cancerous liver cells usually feed on blood from the hepatic artery, while healthy cells are usually fed by the portal vein. Embolization works by injection; a substance is placed in the artery through a catheter. It is possible for embolization to affect healthy cells, so liver function may decrease. However, serious side effects are uncommon.

Chemotherapy is a treatment you may have heard of. It consists of drugs and medications that are designed to destroy cancerous cells. These can be injected or swallowed. Chemotherapy drugs target cells that replicate quickly. The drugs may mistake cells in the bone marrow, mouth, and hair follicles, which normally replicate quickly, for cancerous cells. The drugs are not local, meaning they are spread to the entire body through the blood. This can be helpful if cancer has spread to other organs. However, it can also be damaging since it can attack cells in the aforementioned parts of the body that have not been affected by cancer. Side effects can include hair loss, sores in the mouth, nausea/vomiting, fatigue, bruising/bleeding, and increased vulnerability to infections. These side effects can usually be treated by other medications or by reducing the amount of chemotherapy given.

It is important to note that liver transplant can be an option for liver cancer. This is an option for a small quantity of people, in that very few patients meet the criteria to undergo this procedure. See Chapter 7 for more information about liver transplants.

The ideal method of treatment depends on how severe the cancer is, the patient's overall health, and the size and number of the tumors. Discuss all possible options with your doctor.

PROGNOSIS

Liver cancer has several stages. Each stage defines how widespread the cancer is. The stage of the liver cancer may help determine a patient's prospect of recovery.

Stages

Although not every doctor uses the same staging system, the most fre-quently used is the American Joint Committee on Cancer (AJCC) TNM system. The "T" stands for tumor, and describes the number and size of the tumor(s) present. The "N" stands for nodes—specifically, the lymph nodes—and whether the cancer has spread to them. Lymph nodes are found throughout the body and play a large role in both the circulatory and immune systems. The "M" in TNM stands for metastasize. It describes whether the cancer has spread to other parts of the body.

The "T" groups are as follows:

- **TX.** Tumor size cannot be determined.

- **T0.** No tumor detected.

- **T1.** A tumor exists but has not spread to blood vessels.

- **T2.** Either a single tumor has spread to blood vessels, *or* there is more than one tumor present. However, none of the tumors are larger than 5 centimeters.

- **T3a.** There is more than one tumor present, and at least one is larger than 5 centimeters.

- **T3b.** At least one tumor of any size has spread into either the portal or hepatic vein.

- **T4.** A tumor of any size has spread into another organ or has spread into the tissue surrounding the liver.

The "N" groups are as follows:

- **NX.** Spread of cancer to surrounding lymph nodes cannot be determined.

- **N0.** Cancer has not spread to surrounding lymph nodes.

- **N1.** Cancer has spread to surrounding lymph nodes.

The "M" groups are as follows:

- **M0.** Cancer has not spread to distant lymph nodes or other organs.

- **M1.** Cancer has spread to distant lymph nodes or other organs.

To determine what stage the liver cancer is in, the T, N, and M groups are put together. The stages are as follows:

- **Stage I.** T1, N0, M0. There is a tumor, but it has not spread to any blood vessels. The cancer has not spread to any lymph nodes or other organs.

- **Stage II.** T2, N0, M0. Either a single tumor has spread to blood vessels, *or* there is more than one tumor present. However, none of the tumors are larger than 5 centimeters. The cancer has not spread to any lymph nodes or other organs.

- **Stage IIIA.** T3a, N0, M0. There is more than one tumor present, and at least one is larger than 5 centimeters. The cancer has not spread to any lymph nodes or other organs.

- **Stage IIIB.** T3b, N0, M0. At least one tumor of any size has spread into either the portal or hepatic vein. The cancer has not spread to any lymph nodes or other organs.

- **Stage IIIC.** T4, N0, M0. A tumor of any size has spread into another organ or has spread into the tissue surrounding the liver. The cancer has not spread to any lymph nodes or other organs.

- **Stage IVA.** Any T group, N1, M0. Tumors can be of any size, number, and location. The cancer has spread to surrounding lymph nodes but not to any other organs.

- **Stage IVB.** Any T group, any N group, M1. Tumors can be of any size, number, and location. The cancer may or may not have spread to lymph nodes. The cancer has spread to other parts of the body.

Resectable Stages

The stages of liver cancer described in the section above are the formal classifications. But how does a doctor determine if she can treat the cancer, and if so, using which treatment?

Doctors can classify a cancerous liver as *resectable* or *unresectable.* Resectable means that the liver is able to be operated on or removed by surgery. Most people who are in stage I or II (described on page 65), and who do not have cirrhosis or other severe conditions, have resectable cancer. The cancer can be safely removed by surgery or liver transplant.

Sometimes, the cancer is minor and can be removed, but the patient herself isn't healthy enough and may not be able to tolerate surgery or transplantation. The part of the liver that does not have cancer may have cirrhosis or another damaging condition.

Liver cancer that is unresectable cannot be completely removed. This is because it has spread throughout the liver, or it may be too close to main blood vessels.

Cancer in stage IVA or IVB is considered advanced. It has spread to other organs. In most cases, this cancer cannot be treated.

This section is designed to be a brief overview of liver cancer while looking at liver diseases as a whole. If you are at risk of developing liver cancer or have already been diagnosed with it, see a doctor for more details on the information, treatments, and procedures described above.

HEREDITARY CONDITIONS

Sometimes, liver disease can be caused by an inherited condition. The two most frequent hereditary causes of liver disease are hemochromatosis and Wilson's disease.

HEMOCHROMATOSIS

Hemochromatosis is a condition that causes an excess of iron in the body. It is caused by a mutation in the gene that controls how much iron is absorbed from food. The iron can accumulate in various organs in the body, including the heart, joints, and the liver. If the condition is localized in the liver, the common symptoms are similar to those of other liver diseases, including fatigue, weakness, and jaundice.

The presenting symptoms may vary in different people, depending on which organ is affected by the iron deposition. For example, if there is excessive iron deposition in the joints, then the leading symptoms may be significant joint pain and inflammation. Iron excess in the liver is particularly damaging, however, because if the liver's ability to function is compromised from the iron, it can prevent other nutrients from entering the bloodstream.

Hemochromatosis is thought to be present in one out of every 300 people, although not everybody who has inherited this condition displays symptoms. It is most prevalent in those of Caucasian descent; men are more likely than women to be affected. Hemochromatosis is present at birth, but often, symptoms do not display until about fifty years of age.

As in other conditions that affect the liver, changes in liver function tests can be one of the first signs that hemochromatosis is present. If tests for more common conditions, such as viral hepatitis, prove negative, then further evaluation for other conditions is performed. Because hemochromatosis is a condition of excessive iron absorption and iron deposition, the serum ferritin level and iron saturation level are initially checked. The serum ferritin level is the amount of iron that is stored in your liver, while the iron saturation level is the amount of iron that is bound to protein in the blood. If you have an elevated iron saturation level greater than 60 percent, then it is highly likely that you have hemochromatosis. Further testing is performed to confirm this diagnosis. Specialized genetic testing is usually one of the first tests ordered by the physician if hemochromatosis is suspected. Liver biopsy is done to confirm the diagnosis. An MRI scan can also determine if there is excess iron in the liver.

Hemochromatosis can affect other organs in the body, as well. For example, it can cause *restrictive cardiomyopathy* (*cardio-my-ohp-uh-thee*) in the heart. This condition can present with common symptoms of heart failure, including shortness of breath, swelling in the legs, and weight gain. If restrictive cardiomyopathy is suspected, an MRI showing iron deposition in the heart can be obtained. The principal treatment involves treating the underlying hemochromatosis.

Hemochromatosis generally does not cause long-term damage if diagnosed and treated early. If it remains undetected, the liver may develop hepatitis or cirrhosis. Treatment includes regular *phlebotomy,* which is the removal of blood (similar to the process for donating blood). Removing blood allows you to maintain normal iron levels. If removing blood is not an option for you, a medication can be injected or given to you as a pill. This medication allows iron to be released from the body in urine or stool. This process is called *chelation.*

WILSON'S DISEASE

Wilson's disease (also called *hepatolenticular degeneration*) is a rare inherited disorder, but it can cause liver damage. Just as hemochromatosis is a condition of excess iron deposition, Wilson's disease is a condition that is defined by excess copper deposition. The copper can overload not only in the liver, but in the brain as well; changes in behavior and cognitive function can be some of the first symptoms of this condition.

Unlike hemochromatosis, the symptoms of Wilson's disease appear fairly early in life—between the ages of two and twenty-three. The symptoms are similar to those of other liver diseases, and include fatigue, jaundice, lack of appetite, ascites and edema, cognitive issues (particularly speech problems and a decrease in physical coordination), and bruising. The complications of Wilson's disease can be serious. Cirrhosis may develop because the liver cells form scar tissue in their attempts to repair the damage from the excess copper. The copper sometimes accumulates in the joints or in the heart instead of the liver, which can lead to bone diseases and cardiovascular abnormalities.

Wilson's disease is diagnosed by positively establishing that there is an excessive copper deposition. A physical exam includes checking the eyes; excess copper may deposit itself in a golden-brown ring around the irises, called a *Kayser-Fleischer ring*. One of the blood tests physicians will commonly order is a ceruloplasmin level. Ceruloplasmin is the protein that binds to copper in the blood in order to remove it from the body. A low ceruloplasmin level can be a clue that Wilson's disease is present. Another test measures the urinary excretion of copper over twenty-four hours. There will be an increased amount of copper in the urine of a patient with Wilson's disease. The "gold standard" for diagnosing this condition is a liver biopsy, which looks for excess copper deposition in the cells of the liver.

Genetic testing can also be an accurate indicator of Wilson's disease. Wilson's disease is inherited through a defective, recessive gene; two copies of the gene must be inherited for Wilson's disease to develop. If one parent is a carrier but the other is not, their child will not develop this condition. There are fewer than 20,000 cases of Wilson's disease per year in the United States.

Wilson's disease may cause liver failure if it goes undetected or untreated. As with hemochromatosis, one of the treatments for Wilson's disease is a chelating medication. This type of treatment releases the copper into the bloodstream to be filtered out by the kidneys and eliminated in the urine. Two of the common drugs used for this purpose are *D-penicillamine* and *trientine*. Another medication, *zinc acetate,* prevents the body from absorbing the extra copper from food in the first place. This therapy, however, is more commonly given to children with mild liver disease. In some cases, zinc and D-penicillamine are given together.

One major side effect of D-penicillamine is that it can adversely affect kidney function in some individuals. For example, *proteinuria,* or the spillage of protein in the urine, is a harmful potential side effect. If proteinuria occurs, this is a reason to stop using D-penicillamine. Physicians will closely monitor the kidney function via blood testing and will look for increased protein levels in the urine. Trientine can be used if the person is intolerant to or is unable to take D-penicillamine.

SUMMARY

There are many medical conditions that can affect liver health. In this chapter, you learned more about viral hepatitis, alcoholic hepatitis, non-alcoholic fatty liver disease and non-alcoholic steatohepatitis, cirrhosis, liver cancer, and genetic diseases such as hemochromatosis and Wilson's disease. Many of these conditions exhibit similar symptoms, but they vary in terms of severity and prospect of recovery. Prompt recognition and diagnosis is required to avoid complications and liver failure.

4

Understanding the Complications of Liver Disease

The previous chapters have discussed the various illnesses that can affect the liver, such as viral hepatitis, cirrhosis, and non-alcoholic fatty liver disease. I have also mentioned that when the liver's functions are compromised, the liver is not the only organ that is affected. Recall from Chapter 1 that a healthy liver performs hundreds of functions, such as helping the intestines digest food, clotting the blood, detoxifying the body, and providing nutrients. As you can imagine, liver disease can prevent the liver from successfully performing these functions. Other parts of the body can suffer as a result. In this chapter, I review the ways in which the kidneys, adrenal glands, heart, stomach, and brain work in relation to the liver and how these organs can be harmed in the setting of a liver disease.

KIDNEYS

The kidneys are frequently affected by liver disease, particularly cirrhosis; it is estimated that 10 percent of people with cirrhosis also experience progressive kidney failure.

There are a few ways in which liver disease can affect kidney function. First, the presence of liver disease increases the risk of developing kidney problems due to dehydration. Many people with liver disease often have a decreased appetite, are taking diuretics, and can become very dehydrated if an acute illness (such as bronchitis or an infection) is contracted. Sometimes increasing the dose of a diuretic can raise the risk of dehydration, especially if the individual is also not eating or drinking well.

Second, an underlying kidney problem can be magnified in the presence of liver disease. For example, in someone who does not have liver disease, very low blood pressure or a bad infection (such as the flu or pneumonia) have the potential to compromise kidney function. If this person *does* have liver disease, the degree to which the kidney is affected by the low blood pressure or infection has the potential to be much, much worse.

Hepatorenal syndrome is a condition in which kidney function is compromised due to liver disease. For doctors, this is a diagnosis of exclusion. This means that before diagnosing hepatorenal syndrome, doctors want to first be sure it is not dehydration or another process that is "stunning" the kidneys. These other processes can include infection (pneumonia), low blood pressure, or acute bleeding (common in liver disease). When somebody has advanced liver disease, the intensity of these "insults" are magnified and it can be difficult for the kidney to recover.

One way to describe the adverse relationship that can occur between the kidneys and liver disease is by comparing it to the relationship between the main characters in the movie *The War of the Roses*. In this movie, a divorced couple live in the same house and end up trying to kill each other. This describes what happens to the affected kidneys when they are "living" with liver disease in the same "house": The liver is trying to "wipe out" the kidneys.

It is unknown exactly how liver disease damages the kidneys; the physiologic processes are still being investigated. The portal hypertension (increased blood pressure) that often accompanies cirrhosis may contribute to kidney damage. Conversely, the low blood pressure that is often seen in advanced liver disease also can compromise kidney blood flow and worsen kidney function.

It is important to remember that in the setting of liver disease, the liver's ability to process nutrients and toxins is weakened. To use an example, waste products that contain ammonia can build up in the bloodstream. The buildup of ammonia, which you will read about later in this chapter, can cause increased confusion (hepatic encephalopathy).

Another consequence of liver disease is that it can cause the kidneys to retain excess levels of sodium. When the kidneys' ability to eliminate excess sodium and water is compromised, this can cause edema (buildup of fluid in the legs).

As you may recall, another complication that commonly accompanies liver disease is ascites (fluid buildup in the abdomen). The increase of abdomen pressure caused by the fluid buildup can affect the kidneys in some individuals. Removing some of the fluid (through a process called paracentesis) can improve kidney function because it reduces the pressure in the abdomen.

Aside from edema and ascites, other symptoms of kidney failure include reduced urine output, dark urine, and increased levels of creatinine (a waste product typically filtered out by the kidneys) in the blood. If you already have a liver disease and these signs start to present themselves, this suggests that the liver disease is damaging the kidneys.

Kidney function deterioration that is caused by liver disease is a very serious—and possibly fatal—complication. Symptoms may be relieved by some treatments, such as stopping unnecessary medications (especially ibuprofen, which may increase your risk of sudden kidney damage or failure). If you are taking diuretics (medication to relieve ascites or edema), your usage of them needs to be monitored closely. The excessive use of diuretics may not be well-tolerated if you have advanced liver disease (as they can lower blood pressure) and may have the potential to compromise kidney function. Your doctor will likely be observing you, your blood pressure, and your kidney function very closely. However, if the underlying liver disease is not treated, the kidneys may not be able to regain function.

ADRENAL GLANDS

The *adrenal glands* sit on top of the kidneys in the same way a hat sits on top of someone's head. These glands have two main jobs. First, they help regulate your blood pressure and are your body's fluid managers (i.e., they prevent you from getting too dehydrated). Second, they produce a lot of important hormones, including cortisol, aldosterone, epinephrine, norepinephrine, and many of your body's sex hormones. The roles of these hormones range from creating responses to stress (cortisol and norepinephrine) to regulating blood pressure and keeping your body hydrated (aldosterone) and forming the fight-or-flight response to situations (epinephrine). Whether you have an acute illness or are majorly stressed out, your adrenal glands are producing a lot of the hormones that respond to these occurrences. If you have liver disease, it can affect the ability of the adrenal glands to work optimally. This can cause changes in your emotional responses, heart rate, and blood pressure, along with any symptoms of liver disease that you may already be experiencing.

Several studies have established a connection between cirrhosis and adrenal "exhaustion." It is thought that in the setting of cirrhosis, the adrenal glands may not be working optimally enough to deal with an acute medical condition. They may not be capable of producing the necessary "blood pressure maintenance" hormones (including cortisol, epinephrine, and norepinephrine) that are needed to fight off an illness. These hormones are fundamental to helping the body recover from an acute sickness. Please note that if this "exhaustion" occurs, it is typically only in patients who have to be hospitalized.

In a 2005 study from the journal *Critical Care Medicine*, approximately 350 patients with pre-existing liver disease were evaluated for adrenal insufficiency. This study included four different groups of patients: Those with chronic liver disease; those diagnosed with fulminant (sudden) liver failure; those who had received a liver transplant very recently (within a matter of days); and those who had received a liver transplant within the last six months. The results of the study showed that about 70 percent of all the subjects demonstrated adrenal failure. Of particular note, 92 percent of the patients who had a recent liver transplant (and were being treated with immunosuppressant drugs) were diagnosed with insufficiently functioning adrenal glands.

These studies looked at patients who were critically ill. In Chapter 2, I cited a study that concluded that having cirrhosis is related to a higher mortality in the hospital, especially when someone with cirrhosis is admitted with a serious infection. The liver's inhibitory effects on the adrenal glands' functioning may be one of the reasons for increased mortality (see the example given in the inset "Liver Disease's Widespread Effect" on page 75).

In the event of an acute illness, adrenal insufficiency can be treated with steroids, such as hydrocortisone given intravenously. This "adrenal support" is necessary in order to help the body recover from the illness. In the setting of an acute sickness, adrenal insufficiency can also cause low blood pressure. The intravenous steroids are necessary to help improve and maintain blood pressure.

Adrenal insufficiency appears to be worse in patients who have severe liver diseases; diagnosis and treatment should be administered as soon as possible if this is suspected, especially if an acute illness is contracted.

THE HEART

The blood in your body passes through both the liver and the heart. The liver cleans and processes the blood, and the heart pumps the blood into the rest of the body. The bile that the liver produces plays a large role in circulation by decreasing the hardness of the arteries. A condition afflicting the liver can have a negative effect on the heart (and vice versa).

It is thought that liver disease can affect heart function through several mechanisms. First, it may disrupt the electrical circuitry of the heart. It is the signaling of the electric circuit in your heart that enables it to pump blood (contract) and relax. It is postulated that cirrhosis can affect this signaling somehow; for example, it can affect the heart's ability to contract (*systolic incompetence*). The key to treatment includes optimizing liver function.

One condition that can occur as a complication of liver disease is *cirrhotic cardiomyopathy* (*sir-rha-tick cardio-my-ohp-uh-thee*). This is a recently discovered condition that links cirrhosis to abnormalities in the heart. Symptoms of a cardiomyopathy can include shortness of breath (*dyspnea*),

Liver Disease's Widespread Effect

One of the things you should take away from this chapter is that liver disease affects more than just the liver. If you have a liver disease, your risk of developing kidney disease, heart disease, cognitive impairment, and gastroparesis increases. Risk factors for liver disease, such as diabetes and obesity, affect millions in the United States. Diabetes is also a leading cause of kidney disease, heart disease, gastroparesis, and neuropathy (nerve damage).

Do you see where I am going with this? The organs in your body interact with one another. Chronic illnesses affect the ways in which these organs interact. Together, damaged organs can cause significant disease that is difficult to overcome.

Consider an individual who has been admitted to the hospital with a serious infection (for example, pneumonia). He has pre-existing liver disease and his adrenal glands are not able to adequately respond to the acute stress brought on by the infection, as described earlier in this chapter. Even with the use of medications and supportive measures, it can be very difficult to help this patient get well because multiple organs in his body are so ill.

especially dyspnea that worsens with any kind of exertion. There may be increased edema in the legs, and there can be increased shortness of breath when lying flat (also called *orthopnea*).

A cardiovascular condition called *atherosclerosis*, which is characterized in part by thickened arteries in the neck, may be connected with some liver diseases. Thickened arteries lead to restricted blood flow and potentially to heart disease. Atherosclerosis is caused by plaque buildup in the arteries. This plaque consists of fatty substances, waste products, and LDL cholesterol (the "bad" cholesterol, which is produced in the liver along with "good" cholesterol, as you learned in Chapter 1). Liver disease can weaken the liver's abilities to balance cholesterol levels and filter out toxic substances, which can result in atherosclerosis and other potential heart problems. A 2007 study from the *Journal of Hepatology* linked three chronic liver diseases (chronic hepatitis B, chronic hepatitis C, and non-alcoholic steatohepatitis) to atherosclerosis.

Atherosclerosis typically does not cause symptoms until the arteries become narrow enough to cause chest pain or numbness. Thus, if you have already been diagnosed with a liver disease, be sure to ask your doctor about ways you can protect your heart. Treatment mainly consists of practicing healthy eating and exercising habits. This includes eating food that is low in saturated fat and cholesterol and high in fiber. If you smoke, quitting has been shown to reduce the amount of plaque in the arteries. Taking milk thistle supplements (see Chapter 10 for more information about milk thistle) can help both the heart and the liver, but check with your doctor first before taking it.

Recall from Chapter 3 a condition called hemochromatosis, which is a systemic condition characterized by cirrhosis and restrictive cardiomyopathy. This is not what we are referring to in the above paragraph linking liver disease and heart disease. In this section I am referring to the effects of liver disease of any cause and its detrimental effects on the heart.

Sometimes, heart disease or heart failure may precede the liver disease. One condition, called *congestive hepatopathy*, demonstrates how the heart can play a role in liver malfunction. This condition is so named due to a "congested liver" that occurs when the liver is filled with fluid due to the heart's inability to either pump the blood (*systolic heart failure*) or to relax (*diastolic dysfunction*). This latter condition is the leading cause of congestive heart failure in the United States and can have a severe effect on the liver. Think of it as the fluid "backing up" into the liver because the heart is unable to move the fluid forward. Treatment typically consists of diuretics, as well as medications that can optimize the heart function.

THE STOMACH

Recall from previous chapters that the liver plays an important role in digestion. The liver produces bile to break down the fats in food, and the liver also processes the blood and nutrients that are supplied from the intestines.

Cirrhosis can affect the ability of the stomach to empty its food contents (also referred to as delayed gastric emptying) and it can also affect the movement of the intestines. This is called *gastroparesis* (*gas-tro-puh-ree-sis*). The mechanism by which cirrhosis can cause gastroparesis is being studied, but is not known.

A study from the *Journal of Clinical Gastroenterology* evaluated twenty people who were divided into two groups. The first group of individuals were diagnosed with cirrhosis and experienced symptoms of nausea and vomiting after eating meals. The subjects in the other group were diagnosed with viral hepatitis, but did not have any evidence of cirrhosis. The investigators found that gastroparesis was very prevalent in the group with cirrhosis, while it was not evident in the group of people who had hepatitis. The bottom line of this study is that the presence of cirrhosis can precipitate gastroparesis.

THE BRAIN

As you may have guessed, the brain does not always escape unharmed in the setting of liver disease, especially cirrhosis. I have mentioned in Chapter 3 that hepatic encephalopathy (HE) can occur in somebody with liver disease (particularly cirrhosis). This is a condition in which the brain loses function because the liver is not removing toxins effectively. These toxins, including ammonia, build up in the bloodstream and spread to the brain. In the setting of chronic liver disease, there are many different factors that can cause HE. These range from excessive toxins in the blood to spontaneous bacterial peritonitis (infection of ascites fluid) to drug or alcohol abuse.

Symptoms of hepatic encephalopathy include slow reaction time, poor memory recognition, low attention span, and difficulty concentrating. An abnormal sleeping pattern (sleeping during the day and being awake all night), confusion, and personality changes are signs of progressing HE. In the most severe cases, seizures and coma can occur.

Treatment of hepatic encephalopathy usually includes taking lactulose, which is a laxative, or rifaximin (brand name Xifaxan), an antibiotic. These medications, which you will read about in the next chapter, help reduce the toxin levels in the body. As you will read in Chapter 10, probiotics can also help in the treatment of hepatic encephalopathy.

SUMMARY

Liver disease is not just confined to the liver. It can affect other organs of the body, including the kidneys, adrenal glands, heart, stomach, and brain. Because your liver is central to the digestive system, endocrine system, and other body-wide systems, a disease in the liver can affect how the entire body functions. If you have a liver disease and notice new, troubling symptoms that could signal a complication in another organ, see a doctor.

You may not know that some prescribed and over-the-counter drugs can cause complications in your body as well. In the next chapter, I will cover these medications and their potential side effects. I will also explain the medications that your doctor is most likely to prescribe to you and how these medications can help.

5

Frequently Prescribed Medications

I f you have been diagnosed with liver disease, there are certain medications that have either been prescribed to you in the past or will be prescribed to you in the future to manage your condition. These medications usually treat the symptoms of liver disease (such as excess fluid or hypertension), rather than the liver itself. Although many medications are helpful and can improve your quality of life, other medications (including some supplements and over-the-counter drugs) can harm the liver. With all medications, you should be under doctor supervision and you should use caution when taking them. Liver disease can prevent your body from processing medication correctly, which can lead to further damage and accidental overdoses. The following sections detail the different types of medications and how they can affect your body.

BASICS OF MEDICATION

As you have learned, all substances that you ingest are processed by the liver. This includes prescription medicine, over-the-counter drugs, vitamins, supplements, and herbal medicines, as well as food and beverages. You may be using a combination of these remedies to help your liver recover. However, certain combinations can actually stress your liver further instead of letting it heal. The following sections cover the basics of medication: how to manage what you are taking and ensure that you have all of the information you need about them.

Before Taking Medication

Before taking any medication that your doctor prescribes you, tell your doctor about any medications (including supplements and herbal remedies) you are already taking. Your doctor can advise you on whether it is okay for you to continue your current regimen, or if something you are taking should be removed to prevent unsafe interactions.

Your liver may not be able to process medications normally; side effects of some medications can be magnified if your liver is damaged. Depending on your health and the current state of your liver, it may be okay for you to take over-the-counter drugs (such as Tylenol) without adverse effect. In the setting of advanced liver disease or other conditions, however, your doctor may recommend you avoid such drugs. (See page 90 for information on medications that may injure the liver.)

Do not drink alcohol while you are taking medication for your liver, even if you take the alcohol and medication at different times of the day. Alcohol changes the way the liver breaks down some medications and can cause a buildup of toxic byproducts. The alcohol and medication may fight for the same metabolizing enzymes in your liver, causing the medication to lose effectiveness. Conversely, medication can change how alcohol is processed in the liver; the side effects of alcohol and your level of intoxication may be enhanced if you drink alcohol while taking prescription medication.

Managing Your Medication

If your doctor has prescribed you multiple medications (or if several health care providers are providing medication or supplements to you), you may find that it is confusing to remember their names, what they do, and when to take them. Some helpful habits to establish may include keeping a log of your medications in an easy-to-find place (such as the kitchen table or a bedside stand) or using a seven-day pill container. It may also be beneficial to establish a routine and take your medication at the same time every day.

Your doctor can answer any questions you have about dosages, refills, and side effects. (See Chapter 6 for a list of questions you should ask your doctor.) The medications that doctors most often prescribe to treat swelling and excess fluid buildup caused by liver disease are diuretics (particularly spironolactone) and loop diuretics. I will talk about these further in the next sections. I will also discuss the medications typically used to treat hepatic encephalopathy, high portal venous pressures (high systemic blood pressure), and hypotension (low systemic blood pressure).

DIURETICS

As you read in previous chapters, a complication of liver disease is swelling and excess fluid in either the abdomen (ascites) or the legs and feet (edema) due to portal hypertension. The term "diuretics" represents the medications that manage the swelling; the goal of these medications is to try and eliminate this excess fluid through the kidneys. This is commonly prescribed in addition to a low-sodium diet recommendation.

In the setting of liver disease, different types of diuretics have different therapeutic uses. For example, *spironolactone* (brand name Aldactone) is commonly prescribed to prevent ascites. Another class of diuretic medication, called loop diuretics, includes *bumetanide* (brand name Bumex) and *furosemide* (brand name Lasix). Loop diuretics are used primarily to treat edema in the legs.

■ Spironolactone

Spironolactone (Aldactone) is the best diuretic to treat the buildup of ascites. Health professionals try to prescribe the highest dose of this medication that they possibly can. This is a standard of care for patients who have ascites; it is felt that the higher the dose, the more effective the diuretic will be in preventing the ascites from recurring. Note that this diuretic can also help for the treatment of swelling in the legs, or edema, as well. With that being said, there are potential side effects and precautions that need to be taken into account when this medication is prescribed:

Acute Kidney Failure

Acute kidney injury or failure can occur when using spironolactone. This tends to occur more often in very advanced liver disease than in early liver disease or chronic, stable liver disease. This is because the risk of acute kidney injury increases when you have advanced liver disease, as explained in Chapter 4. Physicians will monitor the kidney function very closely after prescribing spironolactone, and if the creatinine level shows evidence of worsening, they often will either dramatically reduce the dose or discontinue it altogether.

Dehydration

Like any diuretic, spironolactone can increase the risk of dehydration. Dehydration occurs because the diuretics work to push a higher volume of water out of the body more frequently. Signs of dehydration include low blood pressure, dizziness, and dry mouth. You may also notice that you are urinating less. If this is the case, please call your doctor immediately. In addition to being a sign of dehydration, decreased urine output can also be a sign of worsening kidney function.

High Potassium Levels (Hyperkalemia)

Spironolactone is a potassium-sparing diuretic. Potassium-sparing diuretics do not promote the elimination of potassium in the urine, and may therefore cause potassium to build up beyond normal levels. Clinicians will often order follow-up blood work in order to check potassium levels and kidney function. While potassium is essential for your heart to function optimally, too high a potassium level can slow the heart down too much. Think of your heart like an electric circuit; if the potassium level gets too high, it can actually act like a short circuit to the heart.

Low Blood Pressure (Hypotension)

Spironolactone is also used to treat high blood pressure. Therefore, taking this medication can cause low blood pressure (hypotension). The risk of hypotension increases when you are taking spironolactone in the setting of an advanced liver disease, because the liver disease itself can cause low blood pressure.

Nipple Tenderness

Approximately 10 percent of males and a small percentage of females who take this medication develop *gynecomastia* (nipple tenderness). This side effect will go away when the medication use is discontinued. *Eplerenone* (brand name Inspra) can be prescribed in place of spironolactone if this side effect is experienced. Although spironolactone is the top choice of medication to treat ascites (and is less expensive), eplerenone works in a similar method but without the side effect of nipple tenderness.

■ Loop Diuretics

While spironolactone can help somewhat with swelling in the legs, it is mainly used to treat the swelling in the abdomen. A better-suited class of medication to treat edema is the loop diuretics. They are so named because they act in a part of the kidney called the loop of Henle to facilitate a diuresis (an increase in urine production). The most commonly prescribed medications in this class include *furosemide* (brand name Lasix), *bumetanide* (Bumex), and *torsemide* (Demadex). These diuretics are potent, so again, you need to be aware of the potential side effects these medications can have on your body.

Acute Kidney Failure

Dehydration and low blood pressure resulting from diuretic use can increase the risk of developing acute kidney injury. Your kidney function should be monitored closely by your physician.

Dehydration

Loop diuretics are effective in eliminating excess fluid, but they can also increase the risk of developing dehydration. Signs of dehydration include low blood pressure, dizziness, dry mouth, and decreased urine output.

Physicians will watch your lab values closely. Your doctor may ask you to monitor your weight daily at home. If you notice a dramatic decrease in your weight (more than two pounds in two days), please call your doctor; this is a sign that you may be at risk of developing dehydration. Your doctor may need to adjust your diuretic dose.

Electrolyte Abnormalities

Loop diuretics have the potential to cause several electrolyte abnormalities, including low potassium (*hypokalemia*), low sodium (*hyponatremia*), and low magnesium (*hypomagnesemia*). Electrolytes are important in maintaining blood pressure, fluid balance, muscle health, and more. Think again of the comparison between your heart and an electrical circuit. When your potassium and magnesium levels are too low, your heart circuit can become "irritable." Low levels of these electrolytes can increase your risk of developing an arrhythmia (abnormal heart rhythm). This is why your health care practitioner will order blood work, follow your potassium and magnesium levels closely, and replace these electrolytes if necessary.

Signs of low sodium levels include dizziness, cramping, and numbness or tingling. Very low sodium levels and/or an acute drop in the sodium level can cause confusion. This is considered a medical emergency and requires immediate hospitalization.

Hepatic Encephalopathy

If an excessive amount of loop diuretic is used, it can contribute to the development of hepatic encephalopathy (the cognitive decline caused by toxin buildup). This is due in part to the electrolyte depletion described above. The timing of this symptom is important in determining whether the hepatic encephalopathy is caused by the loop diuretic or by the liver disease itself. The following section discusses lactulose and rifaximin, the medications most commonly used for treating hepatic encephalopathy.

MEDICATIONS TO TREAT HEPATIC ENCEPHALOPATHY

As you read in Chapter 4, hepatic encephalopathy is a condition that affects the brain. Toxins that the liver does not filter out build up in the bloodstream, causing cognitive deterioration and personality changes. Two of the most common prescription medications used in the treatment of hepatic encephalopathy are *lactulose* and *rifaximin* (brand name Xifaxan). Both of these work in your gastrointestinal tract to help prevent the buildup of ammonia, a toxin that causes hepatic encephalopathy.

■ Lactulose

Lactulose is a sweet-tasting liquid that really helps in the treatment of hepatic encephalopathy. The recommended dose is usually two tablespoons taken four times a day. Lactulose works by drawing ammonia from the gastrointestinal tract and pulling it into the colon, where it will then be eliminated by the body. It is the top choice of many doctors for treating hepatic encephalopathy. In the United States, it is only available by prescription, but it is very inexpensive and covered by most insurance plans. However, it does have a few potential side effects that you should keep in mind:

Acidosis

Because lactulose is often prescribed for constipation, it can induce diarrhea. An excessive amount of bicarbonate can be lost in the stool, which can cause *acidosis*, a condition in which your body becomes too acidic. (Think of bicarbonate as the body's "baking soda": It is a base that balances out your body's acidity.) If this bicarbonate loss is persistent, your doctor may recommend you take supplemental oral bicarbonate tablets to maintain balance.

Symptoms of acidosis include rapid breathing, headache, confusion, weakness, fatigue, decreased appetite, and feeling nauseous.

Diarrhea and Dehydration

Lactulose is a medication that is often used for the treatment of constipation, in addition to its benefits in helping with hepatic encephalopathy. Doctors want to induce a diarrhea with this medication; that is how they know that it is working. However, diarrhea can sometimes cause dehydration. Your doctor will monitor you closely and watch for signs of dehydration if you are taking this medication. You may be able to increase your water consumption when taking lactulose, unless your doctor specifies that you need to restrict your intake to a specific amount per day because of advanced liver disease.

High Sodium Level (Hypernatremia)

Lactulose can cause a condition called *hypernatremia,* or high sodium levels in the blood. Hypernatremia is due to a type of diarrhea, called *osmotic diarrhea,* that this medication can cause by drawing too much water into the bowels. This can increase the risk of developing dehydration. A lack of sufficient water in the rest of the body causes the sodium level to become unbalanced. Once again, talk with your doctor to see if you should increase your water intake if you are on this medication.

Low Potassium Levels (Hypokalemia)

Using lactulose daily can cause high levels of potassium to be lost in the stool. Many people are on loop diuretics (for the treatment of edema) as well as lactulose; both of these medications together can cause a significant double whammy that lowers potassium levels. As mentioned on page 83, potassium is an electrolyte; if the level is too low, your heart can develop an abnormal rhythm. If you are taking both a loop diuretic and lactulose and your potassium level is dropping, you may need to take a potassium supplement as well.

■ Rifaximin

In some cases of advanced liver disease, even high doses of lactulose may not be enough to treat hepatic encephalopathy. The patient may need to take rifaximin (Xifaxan) in combination with the lactulose to effectively treat the hepatic encephalopathy. Rifaximin is an antibiotic that effectively lowers ammonia levels in the gastrointestinal tract. It is prescribed in pill form.

Some studies have shown rifaximin to be more effective and faster-acting than lactulose. It also has fewer side effects and is generally well-tolerated by patients. However, one concern that many clinicians have with rifaximin is the cost, as it can be very expensive. It is usually prescribed when lactulose does not work on its own or if the patient's body does not tolerate lactulose. Rifaximin is usually taken in divided doses two to three times a day.

MEDICATIONS TO LOWER LIVER BLOOD PRESSURE

If you remember from previous chapters, one of the consequences of liver cirrhosis is the buildup of pressure in the portal vein. This is referred to as portal hypertension. Portal hypertension can have serious complications, including internal bleeding. Medications that lower the pressure in the liver can help increase the liver's life span. The medications that are most commonly prescribed for portal hypertension include *beta blockers* and *nitroglycerin*.

■ Beta Blockers

Beta blockers are medications that can be used to treat a variety of conditions, including high blood pressure, migraine headaches, and essential tremors. Two medications in this class, *propranolol* (brand name Inderal) and *nadolol* (brand name Corgard), are commonly prescribed for the treatment of portal hypertension. Propranolol (Inderal) is usually taken two to three times a day. Many doctors prefer to prescribe a longer-acting form, under the brand name Inderal LA, which can be taken just once a day.

Nadolol (Corgard) is often prescribed to be taken twice a day in divided doses, starting at 10 milligrams and increasing slowly over the entire course of taking the medication.

While these beta blockers are effective in lowering portal venous pressures, there are reported side effects of these medications of which you should be aware:

Depression

Beta blockers limit the body's flow of a hormone called adrenaline. A lower amount of adrenaline can make you feel tired and sluggish; low adrenaline can also be a significant cause of depression. This can be problematic in both the young and old. While liver disease in general can be associated with depression, it is important to note when the symptoms of depression first began. If the depression began soon after starting a new medication, then it is more likely medication-induced than induced by the liver disease.

Fatigue

Beta blockers can cause extreme fatigue, which can overlap with symptoms of depression. Again, liver disease in general is also associated with worsening fatigue, so it is important to note when the fatigue begins.

Hypotension (Low Blood Pressure)

Because beta blockers are used in the treatment of high blood pressure, they work by lowering blood pressure. The doses of these medications are usually increased slowly, but the blood pressure needs to be measured and followed closely, especially in advanced stages of liver disease. Signs of low blood pressure include dizziness and lightheadedness, especially when standing up. If your blood pressure remains very low, you may not be able to tolerate these medications.

Loss of Libido

Loss of libido and decreased sex drive can be side effects of either advanced liver disease or of the use of beta blockers for portal hypertension. This is because of the reduced force of blood flow throughout the body. Again, it is important to note the timing of this symptom to determine what is causing it.

■ Nitroglycerin

If the side effects of beta blockers are intolerable to a patient, some health professionals may prescribe nitroglycerin (*nigh-trow-gliss-sir-in*) instead to treat the portal hypertension. Beta blockers are the preferred medication, however, and studies have not shown a benefit of prescribing these two medication classes together.

Nitroglycerin is commonly prescribed as *isosorbide mononitrate* (brand name Imdur). It is taken orally. The dose starts at 30 milligrams a day and is slowly increased as much as the patient is able to tolerate it. Side effects of this medication can include:

Headache

Nitroglycerin works by opening up the heart arteries and allowing more blood to flow through. As a result, this medication is also used in the treatment of angina (chest pain) and other heart conditions. Headache is a significant side effect of nitroglycerin, especially at the higher doses, because the blood vessels in the head dilate as well. The medication dosage needs to be lowered or stopped if headaches persist.

Hypotension

As with beta blockers, nitroglycerin can also lower the blood pressure; your blood pressure needs to be monitored if you are started on this medication. If the level is too low, the dosage may need to be stopped.

MEDICATIONS TO RAISE LIVER BLOOD PRESSURE

On the opposite end of the spectrum from portal hypertension, one of the possible complications of advanced liver disease is *hypotension,* or low blood pressure. Portal hypertension is a common occurrence in the early stages of liver disease, while low blood pressure tends to be a late symptom of advanced liver disease. Symptoms of low blood pressure can include dizziness and lightheadedness. A medication that physicians may prescribe to help raise the blood pressure is *midodrine* (brand name ProAmatine). This drug works by constricting the blood vessels.

Many people with advanced liver disease have such low pressure that they feel very dizzy when standing up. For some, blood pressure can be so low that they cannot stand up at all. Midodrine helps maintain the quality of life for these patients by keeping their blood pressure at a high enough level to perform basic daily activities.

Midodrine is usually taken two to three times a day. Starting doses are as low as 2.5 milligrams three times a day and can increase gradually to 10 milligrams, three times a day. I usually will recommend this medication be taken at certain times of the day, such as 9 a.m., 1 p.m., and 6 p.m. This is because the effects of midodrine last only a few hours; these are optimal times in which to take midodrine to maintain a higher blood pressure throughout the entire day.

Some people who take midodrine experience an increase in blood pressure when they lie flat. This is a condition referred to as *supine hypertension.* It is more common in patients with diabetes-related low blood pressure, but I tend to ask these patients not to take midodrine any later than 6 or 7 p.m. I also recommend that they try as best as they can to keep the head of their bed elevated at an angle of thirty degrees when sleeping. Consult with your doctor if you believe you have supine hypertension

Medications Given in the Hospital Setting

This chapter talks about medications that may be prescribed to somebody who has liver disease. These medications differ from ones that are given in a hospital. In the event that someone is admitted to the hospital for liver-related problems, many of the medications she had been previously taking may change. If you are in the hospital because of fluid overload and edema, many physicians may switch you from the oral form of loop diuretics to the intravenous (IV) form. In the hospital setting, the IV form of diuretics can be more potent at eliminating excess fluid than the oral form.

If a patient is admitted to the hospital because of acute kidney failure induced by cirrhosis (for example, hepatorenal syndrome), albumin or *octreotide* (brand name Sandostatin) may be prescribed to help protect the kidneys. Albumin is a protein that is given intravenously; several studies have shown that patients with liver disease in the hospital who are given this medication see an improvement in their health and prognosis. Octreotide is also given under the skin, usually two to three times a day.

and have been prescribed midodrine. If supine hypertension persists, it can cause severe complications, such as heart failure or stroke.

The medications described in this chapter so far can be helpful in treating symptoms and complications of liver disease. It is always important to understand the reasons why certain medications have been prescribed to you. Knowing the potential side effects and precautions is important as well. Discuss medications and side effects with your doctor and health care providers to determine which is the best fit for you. Aside from prescription medicine, there are also supplements and herbs you can take to enhance the health of your liver. These will be detailed in Chapter 10. You may also be given a different set of medications should you be hospitalized (see inset above).

When you have liver disease, you need to be extra careful about what you are consuming. The following sections detail medications you should use sparingly or avoid to prevent further damage to your liver. Keep in mind that some of these medications may be perfectly safe for you; it all depends on your current health and the state of your liver. Talk with your doctor before starting any new medication to confirm what you can take and what you should avoid.

MEDICATIONS THAT CAN INJURE THE LIVER

There are several medications—both prescription and over-the-counter—that can adversely affect your liver health. This section reviews the medications you may be prescribed or may already be taking that have the potential to harm your liver.

■ Acetaminophen (Tylenol)

Acetaminophen (widely known by its most popular brand name, Tylenol) is frequently prescribed for the treatment of chronic pain. It can be bought over-the-counter, as well. Even though it is widely available and safe to take in the recommended doses, acetaminophen is a leading cause of acute liver failure in the United States. There are several ways in which acetaminophen can harm the liver.

First, acetaminophen has the ability to cause acute hepatitis. This occurs when taking very high doses in a short period of time. In a safe-dosage situation, the liver breaks down most of the acetaminophen medication and eliminates it from the body via the urine. A small amount of the medication, however, is metabolized into NAPQI, a toxic byproduct that is often produced following alcohol consumption. Usually, NAPQI is removed via the urine as well. When too much acetaminophen is taken, the higher level of NAPQI overwhelms the liver and begins to attack the liver cells.

An acetaminophen overdose can happen accidentally; for example, an individual who is taking a combination of medications may be unaware that one or more of them contains acetaminophen. (See "Are You Taking Hidden Acetaminophen?" inset on the next page.) While it is recommended in the package insert that individuals take no more than 4,000 milligrams of acetaminophen (eight extra-strength or twelve regular-strength pills) in a twenty-four hour period, many clinicians feel that even 3,000 milligrams (six extra-strength or nine regular-strength pills) may be too much to take on a daily basis.

Acetaminophen has the potential to cause liver injuries ranging from benign hepatitis to fulminant liver failure. Those who use acetaminophen chronically (for several months to a few years) are more susceptible to a higher degree of liver injury. Over time, acetaminophen can deplete the liver cells of *glutathione*, which is an important antioxidant that helps maintain the health of your cells. (More information about glutathione can be found in Chapter 10.) At toxic doses, acetaminophen can deplete glutathione in the liver by as much as 85 percent.

Existing liver health is important to consider when evaluating the risk of liver damage from acetaminophen. Some people may not be harmed by acetaminophen at all, while others may be harming themselves without knowing. For example, take the example of a woman with an undiagnosed fatty liver. She is taking between 2,000 and 3,000 mg of acetaminophen a day. Her diet consists of processed food that is low in antioxidant value, which increases the likelihood of her cells also being low in beneficial antioxidants (such as the glutathione mentioned above). The combination of a fatty liver, poor diet, and chronic acetaminophen use has the potential to severely affect her liver over time, even if her symptoms are not severe. You need to be aware of the medications you take and how combining these medications can affect your liver health over time, especially if you have an underlying condition.

Are You Taking Hidden Acetaminophen?

Many people with chronic pain may have multiple prescriptions to manage it. Some of these prescribed medications may contain acetaminophen, even as a secondary ingredient. If your doctor prescribes you any new pain medication, ask if it contains acetaminophen; if it does, you will need to avoid or discontinue taking additional drugs that contain acetaminophen, such as Tylenol.

Common prescription pain medications that contain acetaminophen include Vicodin (hydrocodone bitartrate and acetaminophen) and Percocet (oxycodone and acetaminophen). Both of these medications are often prescribed to be taken three to four times a day. They both are manufactured under many different brand names, which can be confusing. Other common brand names for Percocet include Roxicet and Endocet. Other common brand names of Vicodin include Hycet and Lortab.

The bottom line is this: Read the ingredients (both active and inactive) of the pain medication you are taking before you take it, or ask your doctor if any potentially harmful ingredients are present. The health of your liver depends on it.

■ Antibiotics

Antibiotics are often prescribed to fight bacterial infections, such as strep throat or pneumonia. In some individuals, antibiotics have the capacity to cause liver injury. Studies investigating the link between antibiotics and liver disease have found that it is idiosyncratic, meaning that an adverse reaction cannot be predicted and varies by individual.

Certain classes of antibiotics may have a higher risk of harm than others. For example, penicillin and a class of antibiotics known as the *macrolides* may adversely affect liver function in susceptible individuals. These medications can acutely injure the liver. Macrolide antibiotics include *erythromycin* (brand name Ilotycin), *azithromycin* (Zithromax), and *clarithromycin* (Biaxin)

■ Anti-Seizure Medications

Many of the medications commonly prescribed to treat seizures can have a detrimental effect on the liver. Examples include *phenytoin* (brand name Dilantin), *phenobarbital* (Solfoton), and *valproic acid* (Depakote). Phenytoin, one of the most popular drugs for treating epilepsy, can cause acute and severe liver injury. Phenobarbital is not commonly used anymore, but can have similar effects on the liver as phenytoin. Valproic acid is usually used for partial seizures, but can cause the amount of ammonia in your system to increase (which may lead to hepatic encephalopathy). Note that the amount in the blood needs to be monitored for all three of these medications.

■ Isoniazid

Isoniazid (INH) is an antibiotic medication that is used to treat tuberculosis (TB). While it is effective in treating TB, it has many side effects, including increased liver function enzymes and neuropathy (nerve disease). This is because when isoniazid is broken down by the liver, a toxic byproduct is released. This byproduct can build up over time. If you are on this medication, then your liver function enzymes need to be monitored closely, especially if the dose of your medication is increased.

■ Non-steroidal Anti-inflammatory Drugs (NSAIDs)

Non-steroidal anti-inflammatory drugs (NSAIDs) are a class of medications that include ibuprofen (also known by brand names Motrin and Advil) and aspirin. These are often taken for headache, pain, and fever relief. Although it is a rare side effect, NSAIDs have been reported to cause liver injury. While liver injury due to acetaminophen is often related to overdosing on the drug, liver injury due to NSAIDs is more individualistic and random. With this said, if you are prescribed an NSAID (or take one over-the-counter), you still should not take more than the amount recommended by your doctor or the amount listed on the package insert.

■ Statins

A class of medications called *statins* are among the most prescribed medications in the United States. More than 200 million prescriptions are filled on an annual basis. This number may increase due to changes in the lipid evaluation guidelines (see "Should You Be Taking a Statin?" inset below).

Medications in this class include *rosuvastatin* (brand name Crestor), *simvastatin* (Zocor), *atorvastatin* (Lipitor), and *pravastatin* (Pravachol). Side effects of these medications can include muscle pain or myopathy (a disease that causes muscle pain and/or weakness), increased liver function enzymes, and (in a small subset of patients) memory loss.

The increase in liver function tests is a known and expected phenomenon that occurs with these medications. For example, if you read the package insert for rosuvastatin (Crestor), you will read that there can be elevations in the liver enzymes two to three times beyond the normal range. It is recommended that the individual discontinue or adjust the dose only if the liver enzyme levels elevate beyond three times the normal

---

Should You Be Taking a Statin?

It is important to ask your doctor if you really need to be taking a statin medication in the first place. The lipid guidelines that physicians use to evaluate your risk for developing heart disease changed in 2013. Because of this, it has been estimated that prescriptions written for statins will increase by the millions in the coming years. A few years ago, you may have been found not to need a statin. With the revised guidelines, you may find that you now fit the criteria to be prescribed a statin—even if your cholesterol level is the same. If your doctor is considering prescribing you a statin, it is important to discuss risk-to-benefit ratios first.

ranges. For example, a normal range for the AST (aspartate aminotransferase) value on your blood work is 10 to 50 units per liter. This means a
decrease in or discontinuation of a dose of statin medication is recommended only if your number increases beyond three times this amount
(150 units per liter).

The effect of the statins on the liver is more of a general medication
class effect than the result of taking any particular medication. Side effects
experienced with one of the medications in this class can often be repro-
duced when prescribed other medications in this class. There are alternatives to statins for the treatment of high cholesterol; talk with your doctor
about other possible options.

■ Supplements

Although supplements and herbs (including herbal teas) are often natural, they are not always good for your liver. They are not all subject to the
regulations and tests that prescription medicines are. Some supplements
may have been processed with additives or toxins. Others, such as iron
and vitamin A, can be beneficial in small doses but toxic to the liver in
large doses. If you are seeing an alternative health care provider, you must
let her know if you are taking prescription medications. If you are thinking about buying a supplement on your own, consult with your primary
care physician first. Not every individual will experience adverse effects
when taking a supplement, but it is always a good idea to consult your
doctor first.

The following supplements have been demonstrated to be potentially
harmful to the liver. Note that this is not a complete list:

- Chaparral

- Comfrey (including comfrey tea)

- Iron (more than 45 milligrams a day)

- Kava kava

- Skullcap

- Vitamin A (more than 5,000 units a day, unless it is beta-carotene)

- Some weight-loss products or powders

- Yohimbine extract

SUMMARY

In this chapter, I discussed the medications you are most likely to be prescribed, depending on your symptoms: Diuretics and loop diuretics for ascites and edema, respectively; lactulose and rifaximin for hepatic encephalopathy; beta blockers and nitroglycerin for high blood pressure; and midodrine for low blood pressure. While these medications can be very beneficial in treating the symptoms of your liver disease, they can have significant side effects as well.

Other medications, such as over-the-counter acetaminophen or prescribed antibiotics and statins, can do more harm than good to the liver. It is important to be aware of the medications and supplements that you take, as they can severely impact your liver function depending on your existing liver health. Be sure to discuss with your health care provider before taking any new medication, and always keep track of all medications that you are on. The next chapter will provide you with more information regarding the health care team you will be working with and how to make the most out of your office visits.

6

Interacting With
Health Care Professionals

I n the last chapter, you read about the different medications that you
may encounter. But just as important as the medications are the people
who are prescribing them to you—your health care team. Given the
complexity of the health care system, it is not uncommon for patients to
feel lost and overwhelmed. You may be introduced to several different
doctors and caretakers when you are diagnosed with liver disease. The
goal of this chapter is to help you navigate the world of health care. You
will read about the various members of your health care team, their roles,
and what you can do to maximize your understanding of the proposed
treatment plan for your given condition.

THE TEAM MEMBERS

The health care system is constantly transitioning. In recent years, there
has been an increased focus on a team-based approach to health care.
Liver disease is very complex; depending on the cause of your liver condition, you likely will be seeing several health providers. At minimum,
you will be seeing two professionals: your primary care doctor and a liver
specialist (*gastroenterologist* or *hepatologist*). You may also be advised to see
(or want to consult) other specialists, including nurse practitioners, physician assistants, or dietitians/nutritionists. It is important to be aware of
who these team members are, what roles they serve, and how they should
interact with each other and with you, the patient.

Primary Care Doctor

Your primary care doctor is usually the first person you speak to if you
experience any signs or symptoms of illness. Thus, he will often be the

first person to identify and test for a liver disease. Your primary care doctor has graduated from medical school and finished post-graduate training, either in a family medicine or an internal medicine residency program. It is important to have a trustworthy and comfortable relationship with your primary care doctor.

Gastroenterologist

A gastroenterologist (*gas-tro-enter-alla-gist*) is a specialist in the gastrointestinal (GI) system. You may also know this as the gastrointestinal tract or the digestive system. Gastroenterologists have completed a fellowship in gastroenterology and received specialized training in problems with the digestive system. This includes problems with the intestines, liver, and pancreas. This is the specialist that your primary care doctor will likely refer you to see for further evaluation and management of your liver condition.

As some gastroenterologists have more experience treating liver disease than others, it may be best to call a potential gastroenterologist's office ahead of time to determine if he is the right doctor for you.

Hepatologist

A hepatologist (*hep-uh-talla-jist*) is a physician who has received fellowship training in the liver. While some hepatologists have been trained solely in the liver, others have received fellowship training in gastroenterology as well. Whether you are referred to a gastroenterologist or a hepatologist depends on doctor preference; the gastroenterologist is the specialist most commonly referred to for evaluation of liver issues. Most gastroenterologists often treat individuals with liver disease. But depending on the complexity of what is causing issues with your liver health or in cases where an additional consultation may be needed, you may be referred to a hepatologist for further evaluation and treatment. It should be noted that many hepatologists are located in academic or tertiary care centers. (A tertiary care center provides health care from specialists after referral from primary care.)

Advanced Practitioners

Many physicians—both primary care and subspecialists—work with advanced practitioners, namely nurse practitioners and physician assistants. The people in these roles work closely with supervising doctors, give significant assistance, and can provide you with a diagnosis and treatment. Some people are hesitant to see advanced practitioners; you always have a choice to see whichever specialist you are most comfortable with. However, advanced practitioners are trained and educated for many years and can take on various roles in a gastroenterology or hepatology practice. They can be of great help to you.

Nurse Practitioners (NP)

Nurse practitioners work closely with all types of physicians, including primary care providers and subspecialists. The nurse practitioner has a bachelor's degree in nursing and has pursued additional training, resulting in a graduate or doctorate degree. In many areas of the country, nurse practitioners work independently as primary care providers (in contrast with physician assistants, who always work with physicians). With additional certification, nurse practitioners can become specialists in a certain area, such as gastroenterology.

Physician Assistants (PA)

Physician assistants also work with primary care providers and subspecialists. Physician assistants have usually obtained a bachelor's degree in a health sciences-related field, although this may vary. He has undergone additional training to obtain a master's degree in physician assistant studies. In the settings of gastroenterology or hepatology, PAs can take patient histories, perform diagnostic exams and procedures, order laboratory and blood tests, prescribe medications, and educate patients on a number of conditions. Because the number of specialists can be low, depending on your area, seeing a PA can help reduce waiting time while still experiencing a high level of care.

Nutritionist or Dietitian

The guidance of a nutritionist or dietitian can be invaluable in preventing or treating liver disease. Although these titles sound alike, there are a couple of differences (see "Nutritionist Versus Dietitian" on page 100). People in these positions often work with schools or communities to implement healthier eating habits, but they can also work on an individual basis with patients. In my opinion, nutrition is the backbone of health. Nutrition plays a significant role in maintaining and improving liver health; as you

Nutritionist Versus Dietitian

Nutritionists and dietitians can play vital roles in maintaining your liver health. They can advise you on meal planning and provide you with information about the nutrients you need. However, there is a difference between the two titles. The title "dietitian" is protected by law in the United States; it requires a master's degree and training hours. In contrast, although a college degree is also required to become a certified nutrition specialist (CNS), the title of "nutritionist" can be used by anybody—whether he has formal training or not. Many people who call themselves nutritionists are knowledgeable and helpful; some, however, may not be qualified to give you advice regarding your liver disease. It is best to do some research before selecting a nutritionist or dietitian to ensure you are receiving professional guidance. Ask your primary care doctor if there is anybody he can recommend.

have read in previous chapters, conditions such as non-alcoholic fatty liver disease can be made worse by a poor diet. Even if a liver condition is not caused by a poor diet, eating well can help relieve some of the symptoms. With advanced liver disease, there may be many food and fluid restrictions that you will be advised to follow (for example, you may need to decrease your sugar or fat intake). I tend to recommend a nutritional consultation and follow-up to nearly every patient I encounter in an office setting.

Integrative Health Providers

Some people choose to see an alternative, or integrative, health care provider in addition to their primary care doctor. I prefer to call this "integrative" health care (rather than "alternative" or "complementary") because it is practiced in coordination with conventional treatment. Certain integrative treatments, such as supplements, may interfere with prescribed medication in a way that can cause further damage to your liver. There should always be open communication between you, your primary care doctor and specialists, and your integrative health providers. This ensures that you receive the full benefits of any treatments your health care providers have to offer. (See inset "Communicating with Your Caretakers" on page 101.)

There are many different types of integrative health providers, but they all seek to provide a holistic approach to healing. Examples of integrative health providers can include:

- Anti-aging specialists
- Herbalists
- Homeopathic practitioners
- Naturopathic physicians

In my own practice, I have worked with integrative providers that my patients have been seeing as well as my medical colleagues. It is impossible for one individual to know everything, so it is good to have a "team" of individuals that I can call on when needed.

BEING AN ACTIVE HEALTH CARE PARTICIPANT

In the beginning of this chapter, you read that medicine is undergoing a transformation, meaning that there are new technologies and new means of communicating. These can include communicating with your doctor via email or teleconferencing from your phone or computer. No matter the medium for the interaction with your doctor, it pays to be prepared

Communicating with Your Caretakers

I believe that individuals have the right to see and interact with any health care professionals of their choosing. Getting a second opinion on your diagnosis and treatment options can be valuable. However, one source of concern is when an individual sees an integrative health care provider, but does not inform his other health care providers (such as his primary care physician) or tell the integrative health care provider that he is seeing other doctors. This can be problematic because the integrative health care provider may provide herbs and supplements that can adversely interact with prescription medications.

In the past, I have been surprised by the amount of supplements that some of the patients in my practice were taking. More often than not, I had to "tweak" their supplement and/or their prescription medication regimen in order to avoid potentially dangerous interactions and side effects. Having honest communication with your health care professionals is important—it can only help you.

for that visit. The following sections are all about the importance of an office visit: how to prepare for it and the questions you need to ask to make the most of it.

Preparing for an Office Visit

If you are seeing a physician for the first time, the Internet can be a good source of information concerning the physician or health care provider you are going to see. The Internet also can be a wealth of medical data, although you want to be sure that what you are reading is reliable (see "Using the Internet for Information" inset on page 105). Websites that provide reviews from the public, such as Yelp (www.yelp.com) or Healthgrades (www.healthgrades.com), provide some anecdotal evaluations and patients' assessments of their visits. While sites like these supply you with some useful information, you will be much better off by going from informal word-of-mouth recommendations from people you trust. Ask your close friends or family members about their experience with a particular health professional.

In addition to finding the right doctor, there are some general questions that you may be asked during an office visit that you should be prepared to answer. These questions may include:

- Have you ever previously been diagnosed with a liver problem?

- Is there any family history of liver disease?

- What prescription medications are you taking?

- Are you taking any acetaminophen or NSAID derivatives (such as Tylenol, Motrin, or Advil)?

- What other over-the-counter medications or supplements are you taking?

- Do you smoke?

- Do you drink? If you have quit drinking, how long were you drinking and when did you quit?

- Do you or your family have any history of diabetes or obesity?

While you think about these questions, also consider any signs or symptoms you may be experiencing, such as jaundice or abdominal pain.

Note the timing of these symptoms as well, if you can. The more specific you are, the more your doctor can help treat you.

During the Office Visit

First, understand that an initial office consultation can last, on average, one hour to an hour and a half; follow-up appointments can range anywhere from twenty to thirty minutes. So, it is important to maximize your time with the physician by being efficient and organized.

Bring a pen and notepad or an electronic device with writing capabilities (such as a smartphone) with you to jot down notes and questions. It may also help to bring a friend or family member with you to provide support or ask additional questions.

If you are prepared ahead of time, you can really get a lot out of your doctor visit. Some questions you should ask your doctor concerning your liver health include the following:

What is causing my liver disease?

In many cases, the cause behind your liver disease can be pinpointed, such as the presence of a form of viral hepatitis (see Chapters 2 and 3). Often, however, there are multiple "offenders" affecting your liver function. The most common of these are medications, the overuse of acetaminophen (Tylenol), fatty liver disease, and alcohol abuse. Identifying the cause(s) is key to finding the right treatment.

Are there any dietary changes I need to make?

As I will discuss in Chapter 9, I believe nutrition has a powerful role in the treatment and healing process. Asking about a nutritional consult during your first visit can be beneficial; this can ensure that you get a "head start" in improving your liver health. Even if you have chronic liver disease or cirrhosis—where the damage to your liver may be irreversible— practicing good nutrition may still prevent further complications or total liver failure. Your doctor can advise you on how to adjust your diet to achieve optimal health.

Are my kidneys (or any other organs) being affected by my liver?

In Chapter 4, we talked about the connection between the liver and other organs in the body. A liver disease (depending on the type of disease and how advanced it is) can have severe effects on the rest of the body, so it is advisable to ask your doctor if any other organs are at risk. The kidneys, in particular, are likely to be affected by liver disease, so it is very important to be aware of the signs and symptoms of kidney failure that we discussed in Chapter 4.

What is the status of my liver?

At the end of your office visit, you will want to know (if possible): Is your liver getting better or worse? Do you have chronic liver disease? Do you have cirrhosis? Has your liver function worsened to the point where you need to be evaluated for a liver transplant? Ask about any additional symptoms or complications that you may experience in the future, and which of these require immediate attention. In addition, you should make copies of your blood work to keep in your own file at home. If new blood tests are taken, review the old and new results with your doctor. Be aware that you may be asked by your doctor to fill out a consent form in order to obtain your labs.

What treatment(s) will I need?

In Chapter 5, I described some of the medications that are most commonly prescribed for liver disease. Understanding these medications and how they will work can help you feel more comfortable about taking them. Ask if your prescribed medication is brand name or generic. While brand name and generic versions of a medication have the same active ingredient(s), the nonactive ingredients may vary. There may be a difference between the efficacy of the brand-name medication and the generic medication—different versions work for different people. It is also important to ask about any side effects you may experience, so that they are not mistaken for symptoms. If you are also taking supplements, ask your doctor if they will have any adverse effects when taken with the prescribed medication. Ask about which over-the-counter medications are unsafe to take with the prescribed medication.

These questions help paint a picture of your liver's condition and likelihood of recovering. I cannot overemphasize the importance of having a concrete idea as to where you stand concerning your liver health. Visiting with your doctor should alleviate uneasiness and provide you with information. You should feel comfortable talking to your doctor. If you do not, visit with other health care providers until you find one that feels right for you.

Using the Internet for Information

If you are waiting for your doctor's appointment, you may start to feel curious or anxious about your potential liver disease. The Internet can be a helpful resource for information; with the click of a finger, medical research is readily available online. You can look up almost any health topic, including liver disease. As great as it may seem, there are several issues concerning information on the Internet.

First, you want to be sure that the information you are reading is from a reputable site. Sites such as WebMD (www.webmd.com) and Mayo Clinic (www.mayoclinic.org) are reviewed by medical professionals. The information on these websites tends to be correct and up-to-date. You can also access some articles written by scholars and researchers on scientific databases online, although these articles tend to contain complicated medical terminology. Other websites are not as reputable and may be biased in favor of one view while deriding another. It is important to consider a website's author and source material while researching.

Even if you are using a reputable website, the amount and complexity of the information presented can be overwhelming. It can be difficult to digest and make sense of it all. This leads us to the next problem of the Internet: that of *context*. Realize that not all of the information provided on the Internet pertains to your specific situation. Without proper context, it is easy to start panicking about your health and worry about the worst-case scenario. When searching for information on the Internet, it is key to ask yourself: *How does the information I am reading apply to my own personal health situation?*

How do you begin to understand the context of your own health situation? By speaking with your doctor and asking some of the questions provided earlier in this chapter. The Internet can be informative and can provide you with topics to discuss with your doctor—but it cannot be a substitute for the specific, personal guidance that your doctor can give you.

SUMMARY

If you have liver disease, understanding who the members of the health care team you will be interacting with are and what their various roles are is important. Only by knowing the right questions to ask can you maximize your office visit with your doctor and understand the context of your own personal health situation. Your doctors can provide you with guidance and help you make informed decisions, but ultimately, you are responsible for being an active participant in your liver health. You and your health care provider(s) are a team and should work cooperatively to improve your health.

7

Preparing for a Liver Transplant

I n cases of advanced liver disease, a liver transplant will be considered. During a liver transplant, either a whole liver or a partial liver is taken from a donor (deceased or living) to replace the recipient's diseased liver. A number of factors determine whether someone is eligible to receive a transplant. Your current health status, your age, and how frequently you drink (if at all) are a few of these factors that will be considered when you are undergoing evaluation. The source of your new liver has to be considered as well; you need to be matched with a donor who has a compatible blood type and who is of a similar size to you.

Liver transplants have a high rate of success in treating cirrhosis, chronic hepatitis, liver cancer, and other forms of advanced or irreversible liver disease. However, they also carry some risk of complications. Although undergoing this surgery seems daunting, you will not be alone: There will be a team of several health care professionals who will help you and ease you into this process. This chapter is designed to help you as well, by providing you with the basic information about what you can expect from a transplant. In this chapter, you will read about the tests involved when you are being evaluated for a liver transplant; you will also be given a general overview of the surgery and of the health care professionals who will be a part of the process.

WHO IS EVALUATED FOR A LIVER TRANSPLANT?

There are two general situations in which patients who have advanced liver disease may find themselves. There are emergency cases, in which the patient needs to be evaluated for a liver transplant right away, and (more commonly) there are cases in which the liver function has been deteriorating over a longer period of time. In these cases, the evaluation is considered over time as doctors monitor how severely and quickly the liver function is changing. This latter situation is what we will be focusing on in this chapter, although emergency situations will be discussed below.

Emergency transplants often occur in the setting of acute, fulminant liver failure. This rapidly-occurring liver failure usually results from a patient ingesting a toxin, becoming poisoned, or experiencing an overdose. For example, acetaminophen (Tylenol) poisoning is the most common cause of acute liver failure. In these emergency situations, the destruction to the liver is so pronounced that there is no choice but to bring the patient to a transplant center.

In the more common scenario, a patient with worsening chronic disease has been seeing a gastroenterologist (GI doctor) for a long time. The GI doctor will notice when the liver has worsened to the point that the patient should be referred to a transplant center to begin evaluation. Many of the medical conditions described in Chapter 3, such as fatty liver disease, steatohepatitis, chronic viral hepatitis B and C, and alcoholic liver disease, can bring the liver to this point. The GI doctor will also note the patient's Model for End-Stage Liver Disease (MELD) score (described on page 111) over time. The MELD score is a significant determining factor in the transplant center's evaluation.

THE TRANSPLANT EVALUATION PROCESS

Once your physician or GI doctor has determined that your liver disease has advanced beyond regular treatment, she will refer you to a specialized liver transplant center for further evaluation. The transplant evaluation process usually takes place over the course of a few days and is used to determine your eligibility to be placed on a liver transplant waiting list. Once you are on the waiting list, you begin to accrue time; the sooner you are put on it, the more likely it will be that you receive a new liver in a suitable time frame. The different aspects of the evaluation process are detailed below.

Going to a Dedicated Transplant Center

The evaluation is not done at your physician's office or at your local hospital. Instead, dedicated transplant centers conduct evaluations and perform the surgeries. There are over 100 liver transplant centers in the United States, including some university centers. A great resource for finding more information about a center close to you is the Scientific Registry of Transplant Recipients (www.srtr.org). This organization provides you with a lot of valuable information, including the number of surgeries that have been performed and the survival rates of transplant recipients at specific centers.

It is very important that you be your own advocate concerning the patient care you receive. This means taking initiative and responsibility for your health, especially in the critical weeks before the operation. It also means doing some research when looking at potential transplant centers. There are things you will want to know about a prospective center:

- How many surgeries has that particular transplant center and/or a particular surgeon done in the past?

- How far do you have to drive or travel to get there? (Not every state has a liver transplant center, so you may have to make arrangements to stay somewhere overnight while the evaluation is underway.)

- Does the center participate in your insurance plan?

This last point is important, as a liver transplant can be an expensive surgery; the closest geographical transplant center may not accept your insurance. You will want to choose a center where the surgery will be covered (at least in part) by your insurance company. You will also want to be sure that your insurance will cover any of the prescription medications that you will have to take once the surgery is completed. The medication regimen can be complex, so it will be helpful to have at least some of the cost covered by insurance.

Beginning the Evaluation Process

After choosing your transplant center and making an appointment, it then becomes time to begin the evaluation process. As you are a potential liver recipient, the transplant team's goal during your first visit is to get a vivid idea of you, your wellbeing, and your health habits. The team does this by conducting an in-depth medical evaluation. The members of the transplant team will want to know about any relevant medical conditions and all health concerns. For example, they may ask you:

- Do you have diabetes?

- Is your blood sugar level under control?

- Do you have any heart problems?

- Do you have any history of cancer?

- Do you have any history of breathing problems (for example, emphysema)? If you are an active smoker, then you will most likely not be evaluated for a transplant until you have quit. Tobacco use can actually increase the risk of organ rejection by diminishing the health of the blood vessels.

Expect to undergo a lot of diagnostic testing. The staff at the evaluation center will do some blood work to determine your blood cell counts and your kidney function (if you are not on dialysis). In addition, they will do specialized blood tests that determine your blood type. The tests also allow the staff to analyze aspects of your immune system that will be important to the liver transplant.

In addition to the blood tests, other examinations will be performed. At the minimum, you will be asked to have an ECG (electrocardiogram) and CXR (chest X-ray) done, to ensure the health of your heart and lungs. If you are fifty years of age of older, you may also be asked to undergo age-related cancer screening. This entails a colonoscopy to make sure your colon health is okay. If you are a male, you will be getting your prostate evaluated. If you are female, a mammogram will likely be ordered. Age-related cancer screening is very important in the liver transplant evaluation process. This is because after the surgery, you will be given medications that lower the immune system's performance to prevent rejection of the transplanted liver. Over time, these medications carry a small chance of increasing the risk of cancer. If you have a pre-existing cancer, tests (including imaging studies, such as CT scans) are performed to determine the extent and severity of the cancer. This will help the transplant team determine if you are still eligible for a liver transplant. Each evaluation is personalized.

In addition to the above tests, you may be asked to undergo a stress test and/or cardiac catheterization if needed. A stress test determines how the heart performs both at rest and after stress (exercise) is induced. The stress test is almost standard, as the doctors want to be sure that your heart is strong enough to withstand the surgery. If there are abnormalities on the stress test, a cardiac catheterization may need to be done. A cardiac catheterization measures the pressure in your heart. These tests will be especially important to undergo if you have any history of heart disease. You may be asked to see a cardiologist to "clear you" for liver transplant surgery. Cardiologists can be found in many transplant centers.

If you have any history of lung disease, this has to be further evaluated. You may be asked to see a pulmonologist for more extensive testing of your lung health. Remember from page 110 that if you are still an active smoker, your transplant evaluation may be delayed or cancelled until you have stopped smoking.

The staff also wants to make sure that you have no active infections or hidden sources of inflammation. If there is any active infection in your body, it needs to be treated before you can proceed with any transplant surgery. This even includes undergoing a dental evaluation to make sure your teeth and gums are okay! As you can see, the initial evaluation process for a liver transplant is very extensive.

MELD Score

The Model for End-Stage Liver Disease (MELD) score is a system used by GI doctors and liver specialists to determine the severity of your liver disease. It is one of the most important criteria that is taken into consideration when physicians are evaluating your eligibility for a transplant. The score is calculated using a formula that takes into account a few of the liver-specific blood tests that you read about in Chapter 2.

The following parameters are used in calculating your MELD score:

- **Bilirubin level.** This measures how effective your liver is at excreting bile (the substance that aids digestion).

- **Creatinine level.** This is a test that assesses kidney function. If you recall from Chapter 4, the kidney is often affected in individuals with advanced liver function.

- **International Normalized Ratio (INR)/Prothrombin time (PT).** This is a measure of how effective your liver is at creating blood clotting factors.

In addition to the parameters above, the patient may be asked if she has received dialysis twice in the previous week. The above values are calculated and a score is generated. The scores can range from 6 (mild illness) to 40 (very severe illness); the average score of the patients on the liver transplant list is usually in the low 20s. It is important that testing and blood work be done routinely to have the most updated MELD score available. If your MELD score increases, you may be moved up on the waiting list.

Additional Screenings

If you are undergoing a liver transplant evaluation, your existing physical health and MELD scores (while important) are not the only criteria that are assessed. Your psychosocial health and financial capabilities will also play a role in your evaluation.

The psychosocial aspect is usually conducted by a psychiatrist or social worker. They are looking for evidence that you are mentally aware and well. This is important to the transplant process because the doctors want to be certain that you will follow the directions they give you regarding post-surgery care and medication. If you have a history of harmful behavior to your health or substance abuse, it will not necessarily exclude you from the waiting list; cases are evaluated on an individual basis.

The psychosocial evaluation will also identify the strength of your support system. It is very difficult to prepare for and recover from a liver transplant by yourself. Ideally, you can name at least one person who can care for you during your recovery, keep you on track with your medications, and drive you to and from post-surgery doctor's appointments— not to mention provide you with emotional support.

Financial evaluation and counseling will be provided to you, as well. The ability for you or your insurance to pay for the liver transplant should be secured, but if you are having trouble with this, a case worker can help you develop a financial management plan. It may help to prepare for the evaluation ahead of time by contacting your insurance provider and asking about potential coverage for a liver transplant.

Together with the health screenings and the MELD score analysis, the psychosocial and financial evaluations can help the staff at the transplant center determine your chance of having a successful outcome and a high quality of life after the operation.

Who Will Not Be Evaluated for a Liver Transplant?

Some patients will not qualify for the liver transplant waiting list. This is usually due to the patient having a high risk of becoming ill or experiencing liver failure after a transplant. This can also occur if the patient engages in drinking or drug use, which would damage a new liver. The following people would not be considered for a liver transplant:

- Someone who drinks frequently or is an alcoholic; the individual needs to abstain from alcohol for at least a six-month period before being considered for a liver transplant.

- Someone with a history of active drug abuse.

- Someone who has end-stage organ function (for example, advanced heart disease), for which a person would not be felt to be a suitable surgical candidate. Patients who have end-stage organ function are considered high-risk; their bodies likely will not be able to tolerate the significant stress experienced during and after the surgery.

TYPES OF TRANSPLANTS

There are two types of liver donation: cadaveric donation and living donor liver transplantation (LDLT). Once you have completed the evaluation for a liver transplant, your eligibility for the transplant will be considered. Those who are deemed potential candidates for transplantation are added to a national database developed by the United Network for Organ Sharing (UNOS). Their website, www.unos.org, is an excellent resource for information. The database serves as a "waiting list" of patients who need a transplant.

In addition to providing this database, UNOS also maintains policies for how organs are distributed. UNOS oversees all of the organ procurement organizations (OPOs). There are over fifty OPOs in the United States, each of which represent a specific region and coordinate matches between potential donors and recipients who are in need. UNOS partners with individual OPOs to identify candidates that match the criteria for a donated organ. Factors that determine which recipients first receive a donated liver include the results of the evaluation and specialized testing, blood type, donor age, comparable body size to the donor, and the Model for End-Stage Liver Disease score (see page 111).

Over 6,600 liver transplants, including both cadaveric donations and living donations, were performed in 2015.

Cadaveric Donation

Cadaveric donation is the most common form of liver donation. As the name implies, a cadaveric donation is when a liver is transplanted from a donor who is deceased. A patient who receives a cadaveric donation has been determined eligible to receive a liver after an extensive evaluation. If no living donor is found to be medically able or eligible to provide a liver to this patient, the patient is put on the transplant waiting list to receive a liver from a deceased organ donor.

When a liver becomes available via cadaveric donation, the first patients to be considered are those who are determined to be the most ill within the same local area as the donor. The donor liver is tested for viruses and for compatibility with the potential recipient. The organ is preserved until the recipient arrives at the hospital for the surgery. The liver needs to be transplanted within twenty-four hours after it is harvested from the donor, so recipients must be ready to go to the hospital as soon as they receive the call to do so.

Living Donation

Living donor liver transplantation (LDLT) is a more recently established alternative to cadaveric donation. The first LDLT was performed in 1989. Believe it or not, donors can still be alive when they give a part of their liver to a recipient. Remember from Chapter 1 that a healthy liver has the tremendous capacity to regenerate.

In LDLT, a part of the liver is taken (usually from the right lobe) from the donor and given to the recipient. Both the origin liver and the transplanted segment have the capacity to grow, regenerate, and perform all of the functions that a healthy liver is supposed to do. Both livers will grow to the size of a normal liver within four to six weeks after the surgery.

There are many benefits to LDLTs. For one, the donor is usually somebody who personally knows or is related to the recipient. The recipient's time on the transplant waiting list is reduced or eliminated because the donor is already available and has elected to give her liver to that specific recipient. Less time spent waiting for a transplant means there is less of a chance of the recipient developing life-threatening complications from liver disease. The surgery can be scheduled at both parties' convenience (in a cadaveric donation, the recipient does not always know when the surgery will be and must go to the hospital as soon as possible). A liver from a living donor has a greater chance of longevity and normal functioning in a recipient.

The number of LDLTs has increased in recent years as surgeons and transplant centers learn more about this surgery. Over 300 of the liver transplants performed in 2015 were LDLTs. Many centers across the United States can perform this surgery. An excellent resource for information regarding liver transplant centers and surgery statistics is the American Liver Foundation (www.liverfoundation.org).

Preparing for Your Hospital Stay

After you are placed on the transplant waiting list, you may be waiting weeks, months, or even years to be brought in for the surgery. During this time, you may feel nervous, afraid, or helpless. However, there are some tasks you can do to keep busy and to feel assured that you are ready for your stay in the hospital.

Designate a family member or friend to be your "caretaker" ahead of time. This person will drive you to the hospital when the time comes and will make sure you have everything you need while you are in the hospital. You may want to place another person in charge of taking care of your home while you are away, including retrieving your mail and taking care of any children, pets, or plants.

You will have to be "on call," so to speak, for when a matching donor liver becomes available to you. Stay near a phone whenever you can, because you will have to be taken to the hospital as soon as possible upon receiving the call. A liver taken from a deceased donor can be preserved for up to twenty-four hours. Because of this urgency, you will want to pack a bag for the hospital ahead of time so you can grab it and go. This bag should include a couple changes of clothing, a robe and slippers, your insurance card, medications, toiletries, hand sanitizer or antibacterial wipes, your cell phone charger, some cash, comforting items such as books or music, and a pillow and blanket if you wish. Your caretaker may want to pack her own hospital bag as well. Leave all valuable items at home.

Don't be afraid to reach out for support from your family, friends, caretakers, or doctors—this can be a difficult time, but sharing a laugh or participating in bonding activities can help everybody involved.

THE LIVER TRANSPLANT TEAM MEMBERS

In Chapter 6, I talked about various members of the health care team that you may interact with on your journey to liver health. These include the primary care doctor, the gastroenterologist, and advanced practitioners. In addition to those health care providers, there will be another set who specifically will guide you through the liver transplant process. These include the case manager, the surgeon performing your transplant, the transplant coordinator, and a specialized post-transplant doctor.

The Case Manager

You will likely be assigned a case manager. A case manager guides you through the liver transplant process by explaining to you all aspects of the surgery; providing support during the time you spend on the waiting list; navigating you through the difficult "insurance stuff"; educating you on your post-transplant medications; and carrying out many more responsibilities. She works with the other members of the transplant team to formulate your discharge plan from the hospital. The case manager provides the answers to questions such as: What type of rehabilitation or physical therapy will you need after the surgery? Will this be done at home or in a dedicated rehabilitation center?

The case manager will also work with pharmacists and your insurance company so that you can receive your post-transplant medications. This is vital, as you need to take your prescribed medication when it is needed. The case manager helps you work through the side effects of these medications and emphasizes the importance of sticking to the medication schedule.

The Surgeon

This is the person who will be doing the transplant surgery. She has had many years of experience and training. She sees you during the initial evaluation process to determine if you are a candidate for surgery. Each transplant center is different, but often, the surgeon has a large role in the evaluation process. She also sees you in the hospital after your surgery, and she can see you in follow-up appointments after your discharge from the hospital.

The Transplant Coordinator

Most transplant centers will have a transplant coordinator assigned to you; there is usually someone available 24/7 if needed. The transplant coordinator is often a registered nurse, doctor, or social worker. The transplant coordinator is your lifeline; she is there with you from the very beginning. Not only does she help you balance all that you need to do for a successful transplant evaluation, she also facilitates communication between other members of the transplant team.

The transplant coordinator is also your "care coordinator," especially if you are dealing with multiple physicians. (You will likely be seeing many health professionals who will be involved in your care in some way.) By "care coordinator," I mean that she will help you set up future follow-up appointments, obtain medications, and serve as a resource for any question you may have.

For more information about the health professionals you will interact with, refer back to Chapter 6. All of these different people will provide you with a lot of information, which may become overwhelming. A transplant coordinator becomes invaluable in this case. The transplant coordinator helps facilitate conversations and exchange information between you and your health care professionals.

The Transplant Hepatologist

A doctor who specializes in the liver (hepatologist) will be seeing you after your liver transplant has been completed. This hepatologist may be a different person from your regular doctor or hepatologist. This particular doctor has received specialized training after or during a fellowship in transplant hepatology. One of her main roles is to closely monitor the side effects that your post-transplant medications may have on you. In the first six months following your transplant, you will be taking these medications to prevent organ rejection (by suppressing the immune system) and to prevent infection (because of the lowered immune system).

Every transplant center is different, but usually, the patient can go back to seeing her regular GI doctor after a few months.

THE TRANSPLANT SURGERY AND POST-SURGERY

The surgery itself can take a long time. It typically takes six to eight hours, although in some cases it can take as many as ten to twelve hours. This is a complicated surgery because the liver is taken from one person and given to another; this means that two surgeons are needed (one for each person), as well as additional members of the surgical team (such as anesthesiologists and surgical nurses).

During the surgery, you will be put under anesthesia first. The surgeon will make an incision on your abdomen area in order to access the liver. The blood and bile supplies to your liver will be disconnected so that your liver can be removed. Then, the donor liver will replace the diseased liver, and the blood and bile supplies are reconnected.

You will need to stay in the hospital for several days (possibly a week or more) to recover from the surgery. A living donor will not require as long of a stay in the hospital, but may experience complications or pain. (See inset "Preparing for Your Hospital Stay" on page 115.) The surgery may take longer in a situation in which it needs to be done suddenly. The recipients in these cases are often very ill and require much more critical care-related support to recover from the surgery.

As you recover, you will be following up closely with the transplant team. You will frequently have check-ups and blood work done to evaluate how well the new liver is working. This is then decreased to once a month for the rest of the year.

After the surgery, you will be placed on medications that lower the immune system to prevent organ rejection. Common medications in this class can include tacrolimus (*tack-ro-lime-us*), brand name Prograf, and prednisone. Tacrolimus is a medication that is usually taken twice a day. If you are taking it, you will be asked to have frequent blood work drawn, as the medication's efficacy can be measured via a blood level. Your dosage is then adjusted depending on the blood level. The prednisone is often decreased gradually; most people will be taking 5 to 10 milligrams daily. These immunosuppressant medications have to be taken for the rest of your life to prevent rejection of the new liver.

Possible Complications

As with any medical procedure, a liver transplant may be accompanied by complications. Many of these complications are manageable.

Organ rejection, mentioned above and managed with immunosuppressant medications, is one of the more common complications that occur with a liver transplant; as many as 50 percent of recipients can experience organ rejection in the first month after surgery. Rejection occurs because your immune system detects the "foreign" organ in your body and tries to attack it. Symptoms include fatigue, nausea, abdominal pain, fever, jaundice, or dark urine, although symptoms are not always noticeable. The role of immunosuppressant medications is to relax the immune system's response to the new liver. These help prevent rejection, but usually must be taken for the rest of a patient's life, as mentioned above.

Because of the immunosuppressant medications, another complication that can occur is a high risk of infection. Under the influence of these medications, the immune system's response to foreign matter is diminished, so it is easier to contract viruses (such as influenza), fungal infections (such as Candida), or bacterial infections from the surgical incision. It is important for you to take extra care of yourself post-surgery; this means washing your hands frequently, avoiding people who are sick, eating a nutritious diet, drinking plenty of water, and getting enough sleep at night. Consult with your doctor before taking any over-the-counter medications or supplements.

Complications of the bile duct may occur. Bile can leak out of the duct and collect elsewhere, leading to abdominal pain, fever, or nausea. Or, the bile duct may become narrowed or blocked.

If you experience any unusual or off-putting symptoms after your transplant, contact your liver doctor or general practitioner. An adjustment of your medications may be needed.

Prognosis

The prognosis for liver transplant surgery is generally very good, with about 75 to 80 percent of donated livers working after five years. There are many factors that go into your prognosis, including your age, your health prior to the transplant, and the cause of your initial liver disease.

Your doctor will tell you when you will be able to return to your daily activities. It may take months to recover your full strength, but you should be able to go back to work after about six to eight weeks. You can return to eating your normal diet after the surgery, although it is highly recommended that you adopt a nutritious diet. In rare cases, the original liver disease can recur and another transplant may be necessary.

SUMMARY

A liver transplant becomes a treatment option once your liver disease has reached an advanced stage. Liver transplants are difficult to obtain and costly, but have a high success rate and relatively manageable complications. There is a lot that goes into this process, including a comprehensive evaluation at a transplant center, getting on a waiting list, the surgery itself, and the post-operative care and follow-up appointments. You will have a team of health care professionals and coordinators to support you every step of the way. The information provided in this chapter can help you and your family navigate through this complex and emotionally stressful time.

PART TWO

Complementary Treatment Approaches and Lifestyle Changes

I n the first section of this book, you read about the substances (such as toxins, alcohol, and some medications) that can negatively affect the liver. In Part Two, I talk about just the opposite. The four chapters in this part focus on what you can do to *improve* your liver health. Many of these solutions are best utilized in the preventive and early phases of treatment, but it is never too late to begin a transition to a healthier lifestyle and to become your own care advocate.

Chapter 8 introduces the idea of a liver detoxification plan. You may have heard of a detox before—but it is often associated with a fast "cleanse," which can do more harm than good. In this chapter, I suggest instead a *slow* detox plan that places an importance on a balanced diet. The goal of a detox is to refresh and "reset" the liver and strengthen its reserve against toxins. This chapter emphasizes that you do not have to restrict food to eliminate toxins from your liver.

In Chapter 9, I discuss the "liver-based nutrition program." The idea behind this nutrition program is that it is a long-term way to maintain a healthy liver. This can prevent a mild liver disease from further develop-ing, and can preserve the functions of a liver that is afflicted with a more advanced condition. I go over the basic macronutrients (such as fats, carbohydrates, and protein) and explain how much of each you should consume. I also review some common and popular diets that could be helpful in your wellbeing. While you should always consult with a doctor before overhauling your diet, this chapter lays the groundwork for a discussion.

In Chapter 10, the focus is placed on supplements and herbs that are valuable to liver health, but have benefits in other parts of your body, as well. These supplements include certain antioxidants, vitamins and minerals, and probiotics. They work together with a nutritious diet to give your liver a boost and protect it from harmful substances. This chapter serves as a guide you can reference when talking with your doctor about your treatment options.

Chapter 11 discusses the importance of exercise and how to develop an exercise plan that works for you. You may find it difficult to start exercising when you have a liver disease, but even thirty minutes of activity a day is enough to improve your overall health. Exercise is especially helpful if you have fatty liver disease, high blood sugar, high cholesterol levels, or muscle weakness due to advanced liver disease. Combined with a healthy diet, exercise can reduce the incidence of obesity, which is the most common cause of fatty liver disease.

While Part One provided you with the information you need to know about the liver and its diseases, Part Two gives you the strategies and tools you can use to take your liver health into your own hands. Together with your health care providers, you can create a customized treatment plan that best benefits you.

8

Developing a Liver Detoxification Plan

R ecall from Chapter 1 that the liver is the body's chief processor and toxin remover. We are surrounded by toxins every day, even if they are not always visible. Think about the processed foods, pesticides, and chemicals that we are either exposed to or are putting into our bodies on a daily basis. Then, add any preexisting conditions, such as diabetes, fatty liver, chronic acetaminophen use, or alcoholism, and you can see that the liver fights a lot of battles on a daily basis.

Depending on how exposed your liver has been to toxins, there may be a significant need for you to undergo a detoxification process. *Detoxification* is the process of eliminating toxic substances from the liver, and therefore cleansing the rest of the body. It is done by modifying nutritional habits and using supplements in order to make full use of the liver's naturally existing detoxifying and metabolizing properties. It sounds like a play on words, but it may be necessary for some people to detoxify the organ that is already the "major detoxification system" of their bodies.

In this chapter, I will discuss the purpose of detoxification and the basic components of this process. But before we delve into detoxification any further, you first need to ask yourself (and your doctor): "Am I a candidate for a liver detox?" The answer depends on your age, active health issues, medications you are taking, and the status of your liver health (i.e., if you have a mild or an advanced condition).

Before initiating any detoxification plan, be sure to speak with your doctor or health care professional. If you have an advanced condition, such as cirrhosis, your liver may not be able to handle the effects of detoxification, no matter how "light" the process is.

DEFINING A TOXIN

You may be wondering, "What exactly is a toxin, anyway?" Toxins are materials that linger in the body and cause or aggravate illness. Toxins include obvious culprits such as alcohol, illegal drugs, pesticides, industrial chemicals, aerosol sprays, bisphenol A (BPA), cigarette smoke, and factory pollution—but they can also be found in medications, food additives, and even materials produced by the body itself as it digests and metabolizes what we consume. These toxins produced by the body are called *endogenous toxins,* and include substances such as carbon dioxide, ammonia, and bacteria. Toxins from outside the body are called *exogenous toxins.*

We unknowingly ingest toxins every day, whether we are placing them on our skin, eating them, or breathing them in. According to the Environmental Protection Agency, over 4 billion pounds of toxic waste were released into the environment in 2014. That is just in one year—over time, it really adds up.

Signs of Toxin Buildup

I have mentioned before that the liver's main role is to detoxify the body. But when you have liver disease, the ability of the liver to process and eliminate toxins can be slowed. How do you know if your liver is not adequately removing toxins from your body on its own?

When toxins build up in your body, key nutrients and antioxidants (such as glutathione) become depleted. There is an increase in free radical formation, which causes *oxidative stress* on the hepatocytes (liver cells). Oxidative stress is an imbalance in the body that affects its ability to repair damage. Toxin buildup can prevent the liver's detoxification pathways from performing optimally and eliminating these damaging free radicals. Chronic illness is a consequence of toxin buildup. Physical signs of buildup can include fatigue, weakness, confusion, headache, dizziness, difficulty sleeping, and abdominal discomfort. These can occur in anyone who has had toxin exposure, even if they do not develop liver disease.

The following factors increase your risk for toxin exposure and buildup:

- Being dehydrated. Drinking more water helps the kidneys filter toxins out of the body.

- Constipation or infrequent bowel movements (toxins can form in the bowel).

- High drug, alcohol, or medication intake. (This does not mean you should stop taking your medications. It simply means you should be aware of the potential effects your medications can have on the liver—refer back to Chapter 5.)

- Lack of exercise (exercise promotes the elimination of toxins).

- Living or working on a farm that uses pesticides; eating food from farms that use pesticides.

- Living or working in a building that is heavily exposed to toxic substances (i.e., is constructed of synthetic materials, is often cleaned with strong chemicals or aerosols, has undergone fumigation or pest control, etc.).

If you are frequently exposed to these risk factors, a detoxification plan can be very beneficial. Part of the goal of detoxification is to provide the cells with much-needed nutrients; the cells use these nutrients to repair, regenerate, and remain viable.

Why Detox?

Given that the liver is exposed to so many stressors, the question arises: Is there ever a need for liver detoxification? Most of the time, the answer is yes. There is no doubt about the effects that long-term toxin exposure has on the body, the prime examples being chronic illness, diabetes, and obesity. Your liver has different processes of detoxification.

I believe that food and supplements can be used to optimize the efficiency of the various detoxification pathways of the liver. An article from the *Journal of Nutrition and Metabolism* discussed the positive effects that food and nutrients can have on the liver. I will provide an example:

Glutathione S-transferase (GST) is a potent detoxification enzyme in the liver. Green, cruciferous vegetables such as kale, broccoli, and Brussels sprouts, as well as garlic and onions, can increase the activity level of GST (which is a good thing). Other supplements, including turmeric, resveratrol, and fish oil, also increase the efficiency of this enzyme. These vegetables (and other foods and supplements) are a staple of many detoxification programs.

BEFORE YOU BEGIN

It is very important to note that I do not recommend starting a detoxification plan on your own without appropriate medical supervision. You and your health care provider(s) need to take any other medical conditions into account before starting a detox. There are many conditions and medications, described in the following sections, that can interfere with the safety and efficacy of a detox plan.

Once you have talked with your doctor (and he is on board with your initiating a liver detox plan), you then need to start "checking in" with him on a regular basis. Depending on any pre-existing conditions, you may need to keep a list of your blood glucose levels or blood pressure measurements and see what medications need to be adjusted or even temporarily stopped. Blood work may need to be done to monitor your electrolyte and mineral levels (these include sodium, potassium, magnesium, calcium, and vitamin D), as well as your liver and kidney function. This is important because the blood work can identify any significant nutrient deficiencies. The blood work can also determine if you need to modify some of the specifics of your detox plan. As you develop the dietary portion of your detox plan, it can be especially helpful to connect with a nutritionist or dietitian (if you have the opportunity to do so).

A detox is mainly recommended for those who have a history of unhealthy dietary or health habits; a detox allows them to "reset" their bodies and livers by "starting over." If your diet is such that you are eating more of a plant-based, organic, high-fiber diet, and supplementing with certain nutrients (discussed in Chapter 10) on a regular basis, then you are doing all that you can to provide your body and liver with the nutrients they need. In this case, a liver detox may not be necessary.

I would not advocate a detox plan for the following groups of people, as well:

- Those who have been diagnosed with cirrhosis or another advanced liver disease.

- Those who have been diagnosed with kidney disease or who have been told they have kidney problems. In this scenario, I worry that the kidneys would not be able to handle the stress of a detox.

- Those who have an underlying heart condition, such as coronary disease or a history of congestive heart failure.

- Those who have diabetes; the risk of low blood glucose levels, or hypoglycemia, is too significant. This is very important and is discussed further in the section "Diabetes and Detox" below.

- Those who are taking warfarin (brand name Coumadin) or other blood thinners. The blood level measurements of these medications as well as their effectiveness can be influenced by certain foods, especially large amounts of certain vegetables, which (as you can guess) are an important part of any detox program.

The bottom line is this: *You need to consider your other health conditions as well as the medications you are already taking before you can start a detox plan. Safety is important, and this is why I emphasize having an open and honest discussion with your physician. It is important to review your medication list and discuss what medications need to be continued, what can be stopped, and what medications need to have their dosages adjusted.*

Diabetes and Detox

If you have diabetes, it is particularly risky for you to begin a detoxification process. Let's say that you have been told by your doctor that your liver health is okay, and you proceed to begin a detox. One important component to detoxification is modifying your food consumption, which might lower your blood glucose levels. Perhaps you are taking insulin or other medications that already lower your blood glucose levels. You will need to speak with your physician to either adjust or even temporarily discontinue your medications in order to avoid hypoglycemia (low blood glucose levels). The insulin dose may have to be reduced. If you have diabetes and decide to undergo detoxification, then you need to monitor your blood glucose levels at least twice a day (if not more) during your detox.

If you are diabetic and are starting a detox, you should always carry some food, such as hard candy or graham crackers, on you to eat in case your blood glucose gets too low. You also should carry an emergency glucagon kit (which can temporarily raise blood glucose levels when injected). However,the bottom line is that even with these precautions, I strongly recommend that anyone with diabetes does not undergo liver detoxification because the risk of hypoglycemia is too high.

Blood Thinners and Detox

If you are taking blood thinners, then a liver detox program may not be the best idea for you. As noted on page 127, the vitamin K content in green, cruciferous vegetables (e.g., kale and broccoli) can decrease the efficacy of blood thinners. These vegetables are a staple of a detoxification.

There are meters that you can purchase to check your prothrombin time and INR (International Normalized Radio), to measure how thin your blood is, at home. These meters usually are covered by Medicare and most insurance companies, but even so, it is my opinion that a liver detox program is too risky to undertake if you are on a blood thinner.

Blood Pressure Medications and Detox

High blood pressure is often present in those with liver disease. Many people take blood pressure medications as a result. High blood pressure is associated with a high sodium intake and, more significantly, a high sugar intake (some recent studies have shown that ingesting sugar drives inflammation and high blood pressure). This is important to note because during a detox, the foods that are often recommended are low in salt and sugar. If you are sensitive to the amount of salt you take in, the combination of a restricted salt intake plus the effect of the blood pressure medications may cause a serious drop in your blood pressure (hypotension). Likewise, if your sugar consumption is dramatically restricted, this can lower your blood pressure as well. If you have high blood pressure and decide to undergo a liver detox, you need to check your blood pressure on a daily basis.

Although it is not as common as high blood pressure, in some cases of advanced liver disease, low blood pressure can occur. If your blood pressure is very low to begin with, I would advise against starting a detox plan because your blood pressure may drop to a dangerous level.

When to Stop Detoxification

You may "feel bad" in the first few days of a detoxification process. This is to be expected; the toxins, which have remained in the liver for so long, are now entering the bloodstream to be eliminated. The inflammatory reaction that follows is called the *Jarisch-Herxheimer reaction*. This reaction may cause you to have flu-like symptoms and to feel feverish and fatigued. It should dissipate after a few days to a week.

If you find you need to stop following a detoxification program, it is okay to stop no matter where you are in the process. Signs that you need to end the detox process include:

- Dizziness or lightheadedness

- Persistent abdominal cramping and/or diarrhea

- Persistent flu-like feeling that continues after the first few days of starting the detoxification

- Persistent nausea or vomiting

- Persistent weakness or fatigue

- Shortness of breath or chest pain (this is rare; however, be aware that it is still a possible side effect)

If you do intend on pursuing a detox, I recommend a "slower," more gradual process (see page 132), which greatly minimizes the risk of developing these side effects. The slow detox places an emphasis on nutrition and should be able to be completed without a concern.

THE PROCESS: FAST VERSUS SLOW

Once you have been cleared by your health care provider, you can begin your detox. However, there is so much information about detox plans in books and on the Internet that you may not know where to begin.

You may have heard of "fast" detoxifications and "slow" detoxifications. Fast plans are advertised to "cleanse" your body over a short period, usually a few days. A "colon cleanse" is a popular example of a fast detox. I believe that these fast plans are too intense for someone with liver disease to handle, especially if he also has kidney disease. The slower detoxification that I recommend takes place over a few weeks with a gradual taper and transition into a long-term or lifelong nutrition plan.

Below are some more details on the slow detoxification.

Initial Phase and Maintenance Phase

The slow liver detox plan takes place over four to six weeks. There are two basic aspects: the *initial phase* and the *maintenance phase*. The initial phase, lasting one to two weeks, is the beginning phase; it tends to be more restrictive in terms of what you can eat, as the goal is to enhance elimination of the toxins. The maintenance phase, meanwhile, tends to be less restrictive as you become healthier and "toxin-free." The maintenance phase of the detox lasts for the next four weeks. After that, the detox is finished; however, it should ideally result in a long-term lifestyle change that allows you to continue receiving the benefits of a detox.

The main difference between the initial phase and the maintenance phase is that during the initial phase, there is a significant emphasis on hydration, consumption of antioxidant-based supplements, and increased use of plant-based protein shakes. During the initial phase, it is crucial that you maintain your nutrient needs, as the symptoms of acute detoxification (see page 129) can occur during this time. In addition, the liver and kidneys require significant nutritional support. When you begin a detox program, the toxic load that is to be eliminated can be significant. You need to stay hydrated, as the kidneys will be working to excrete the toxins from your body.

Hydration

Although the risk of dehydration is lower during a slow detox than a fast detox, it is still essential to be hydrated throughout the process. You need to maintain hydration with at least six to eight glasses of water a day, unless there is a reason for you to be fluid-restricted. Water is fundamental to flushing the toxins out. I personally am a fan of lemon water and alkaline water, in particular. Alkaline water has components added to it to make it less acidic than regular water. Studies suggest that alkaline water is bone-protective, as well as a promoter of gut health and motility.

In addition to drinking alkaline water throughout the day, you can supplement with other liquids high in antioxidant activity, such as green tea. Juices or smoothies can be added, as well. I would refrain from consuming caffeine during the detox because it has a diuretic effect; the goal is to keep the organs, especially the kidneys, hydrated as you detox. Avoid sugar-sweetened packaged juices and carbonated soft drinks.

Juicing

Juicing is a delicious and healthy way to provide your body with the nutrients it needs. Many juicers can be purchased for under $100. I recommend juicing fruits that are lower on the glycemic index, such as apples or blueberries. Mixing these fruit juices with juice from vegetables (such as broccoli and kale) gives your body a much-needed antioxidant load, and also counters the symptoms of acute detoxification you read about earlier in the chapter. In addition to the six to eight glasses of water you are consuming, one to two eight-ounce glasses of juice can be beneficial.

Supplements

There are certain supplements that I recommend using during the liver detoxification process because they provide much-needed nutrients and antioxidant support to the liver. These include:

- **Alpha-lipoic acid.** This is an antioxidant that has been shown to play a beneficial role in metabolism. It has also been found to have properties that protect against fatty liver disease and high triglyceride levels. However, it can lower blood glucose levels. Given that there is already a likelihood of having low blood glucose levels during the detox process, I prefer to wait a few weeks before adding this supplement to a patient's detox program. As I mentioned on page 127, patients who are prone to low blood glucose levels should check these levels every day while on a detox plan. If these levels tend to be low, it may not be safe to take alpha-lipoic acid. During the initial one to two weeks of the detox plan, taking 200 milligrams twice a day is not bad to start. Some people may get mild nausea or stomach upset with this supplement, which may persist. If that is the case, simply stop taking it. During the maintenance phase, decrease the dose to 200 milligrams once a day.

- **Milk thistle.** Milk thistle is an herbal supplement that has been used for thousands of years to treat liver problems. Take at least 200 milligrams twice a day to provide tremendous support to the liver during the initial phase. Given this herb's potency when it comes to liver protection, I would maintain the same dose during the maintenance phase as well.

- **N-acetylcysteine.** This supplement replenishes glutathione, which is the "chief antioxidant" in the liver, and is therefore very important. You may take 600 to 1,200 milligrams twice a day, every day for the first one to two weeks. After the initial phase, decrease this dose to once a day.

- **Probiotics.** Probiotics provide your intestines with "good" gut bacteria to help digest your food and counteract "bad" bacteria. To maintain a healthy gastrointestinal tract and liver, I recommend taking a probiotic twice a day during the first two weeks (or as tolerated; it may cause loose stools in some people) and at least daily during the maintenance phase.

- **Selenium.** This is a very helpful, liver-friendly nutrient. It has anti-inflammatory and immune system-protecting qualities. Dosages of 50 to 100 micrograms daily are recommended. Do not take more than 400 micrograms a day. Selenium can interfere with medications, such as statins, so check with your doctor before adding a selenium supplement to your routine.

- **Vitamin B.** A good vitamin B supplement that is high in thiamine, folic acid, pyridoxine (vitamin B6), and cobalamin (vitamin B12) is essential. The liver utilizes these vitamins for its daily functions. This should be taken daily during both the initial and the maintenance phases. Along with probiotics and milk thistle, I believe a good B vitamin complex is essential to take at least two or three days a week even after the detox has been completed.

See Chapter 10 for more information regarding supplements.

AN EXAMPLE OF A DETOX PROGRAM

The following outline for a slow detoxification is based on my own experiences and teachings. Talk with your doctor about what the best detox plan is for you.

Initial Phase

Breakfast. During the first one to two weeks of the detox, you will begin your day with an eight-ounce glass of lemon water. Then, on alternating days, you will drink either a plant-based protein and fiber drink or a fruit and vegetable juice for breakfast.

The drink that I make in the morning consists of two scoops of a plant-based protein powder, which contains about 20 grams of protein, all of the amino acids (including leucine and the branched chain amino acids), high omega-3 fatty acid content, and positive health effects from the plant extracts (e.g., kale, spirulina, and broccoli). I add powdered fiber to this and mix it all in an eight-ounce glass of water. I would try and drink this every other day (e.g., Sunday, Tuesday, Thursday, and Saturday).

On the other days, switch this drink for a fruit and vegetable juice. Try to use fruits lower on the glycemic index (i.e., that do not raise your blood glucose levels too much). For example, one of my favorite juicing recipes includes kale, carrots, and broccoli, while adding apple for flavor and fiber. Add cinnamon for flavor and voila! When juicing, you can experiment according to your own personal preferences, but I advise that you use a higher number of vegetables than fruit.

If you are still hungry mid-morning, you can carry around apple slices or vegetable slices (e.g., carrots) to carry you through to lunch.

Lunch. For lunch (about 11 a.m. or 12 noon), nothing is better than a salad. During the one to two week-long induction phase, lunch is going to be your main meal. Get passionate about your salad. Add all kinds of leafy greens and vegetables. Use olive oil and vinegar for your dressing. You can add a half-cup of a protein source such as salmon, tuna, or chicken to make the salad more filling. Drink an eight-ounce glass of lemon water with this meal.

Dinner. For dinner, have a plant-based protein shake mixed in an eight-ounce glass of water (the same one that you make for breakfast).

At approximately 8 p.m., drink another half-scoop of your protein powder in a shake.

Throughout the day, drink multiple six-to-eight-ounce glasses of water. You can also make a juice once or twice during the day to provide you with antioxidant support.

After you have completed this program for one to two weeks, reassess how you feel and where you are. If you are ready, you can then begin to go onto the maintenance aspect of this program.

Maintenance Phase

During the four-week maintenance phase, I would decrease the dosage of most supplements by 50 percent. If you find it difficult to maintain the same degree of hydration that you did during the initial phase, you can decrease the frequency of hydration by one-third. However, if at any time you feel dehydrated, drink water immediately.

During the maintenance phase, the goal is to consume four small meals a day. Breakfast can be expanded to be (for example) whole-grain cereal topped with berries one day, and egg whites the next day (these are a good source of protein). If you miss a meal due to work or a busy schedule, you need to drink a plant-based protein shake to replace it. The other "rules" during this phase are that at least one main meal each day needs

A Note About Exercise

Exercise is an important component of any detox program and long-term nutritional plan. Exercising promotes the elimination of toxins through the skin, an organ that plays a vital role in detoxification. During the initial phase of a detox, you should do only mild exercise every day to start. This can be as simple as taking a brisk walk. Movement is important, but I would not start out with intense exercise the first week or two upon starting your detox plan. If you feel okay during the maintenance phase, you can increase the intensity of your exercise to work up a sweat. Again, any type of exercise is good; it is important not only for the detox process, but also for maintaining a healthy liver for the rest of your life. (See Chapter 11 for more about the benefits of exercise.)

to be salad-based. If a meal includes fish, chicken, turkey or tuna, you need to have two vegetable servings with it.

The goal of this aspect of the detox plan is to make the transition to a cleaner way of eating in your everyday life. You can also begin to incorporate more exercise (see inset above).

In all phases of a detoxification process, the food should be organic (if possible), because organic food does not use pesticides. Avoiding food that is high in sugar or salt is key. (See Chapter 9 for more information on diet.)

SUMMARY

Implementing a liver detoxification plan can be a medication-free way of improving your liver and overall health, especially if you follow a slow detox plan over a course of four to six weeks. The slow detox can then transition into a broader, lifelong nutrition plan. The goal of a detox is to eliminate the harmful substances we unknowingly take in on a daily basis. Supplements can be used to enhance your program.

For your own safety, there are many precautions that you need to take prior to initiating a detox plan. It is very important to check in with your doctor and other health professionals on a regular basis. They need to be part of the process of detoxification, as it can affect many organs of the body. Safety comes first before anything else.

9

Creating a Liver-Based Nutrition Plan

In the previous chapter, I talked about the components of a liver detox-ification program. However, you may not be medically cleared for a detox, whether it is because of your current health or the medications you are taking. You simply may not want to undergo a detox. You still have options for improving your liver health without having to commit to a detox; one of the key aspects of treating liver health is nutrition. Food has the power to harm (poor dietary habits can contribute to heart disease and diabetes), but food also has the power to heal. It is all about eating the right foods, and eating the right amount of them. A healthy nutrition plan can benefit your liver and body in countless ways—and when you are eating healthy, there is less of a need to consider a detoxification process. Many foods naturally provide you with important vitamins, min-erals, and antioxidants.

The degree of malnutrition that exists in individuals with liver disease is often underestimated. Someone who is obese may seem "well-fed," but may actually have severe nutritional deficiencies that can aggravate liver disease. Gaining an understanding of your dietary needs is vital to your health, wellbeing, and life.

In this chapter, I discuss various food options and how to develop a liver-specific nutrition plan. The idea behind a "nutrition-based plan" is that it is going to be a long-term, ongoing habit. This is in contrast to a temporary "diet" (e.g., "If I follow this diet for ten days, I will lose weight and be healthy"). For simplification purposes, the term "diet" will be used in this chapter to signify the nutrition-based plan.

THE IMPORTANCE OF EATING RIGHT

One of the liver's most important functions is processing nutrients. This includes converting fats and amino acids into energy; regulating the amount of sugar in your blood; processing proteins to build muscles; and storing minerals, such as iron, for later use.

While the liver is important for nutrition, the reverse is true, as well: What you eat can help or harm your liver. Since everything you consume is processed in the liver, having large amounts of certain substances can damage the liver over time.

A good nutrition plan is beneficial not just for the liver, but also for the other organs that the liver interacts with, such as the heart and the kidneys. In this chapter, you may notice that the beneficial components of the liver nutrition plan can overlap and benefit other organs in the body and the body as a whole.

While poor nutrition is usually not the sole cause of liver disease (with the exception of diseases caused by excessive alcohol consumption), a consistently poor diet certainly does not help. Eating a healthy, balanced diet, on the other hand, can slow or possibly prevent further liver damage. But what constitutes a balanced diet? In the following sections, I will review components found on every nutrition label—calories, carbohydrates, cholesterol, fat, protein, sodium, and vitamins and minerals—and discuss the appropriate amounts of each, depending on how advanced your liver disease is.

NUTRITION PLAN COMPONENTS

Before changing your diet, it is important to first know the state of your liver's health. Do you have risk factors for liver disease, but have not been diagnosed with one? Have you been told that you have a sudden and acute illness, or a stable and chronic one? Do you have cirrhosis?

If you have cirrhosis or advanced liver disease, your nutritional needs are going to be a little different than if your liver is still functioning effectively. Remember that cirrhosis is scarring of the cells, meaning that they do not have the capacity to regenerate as they would in a healthier liver. A balanced and focused nutrition plan may boost the efficiency of the liver cells, helping to prolong the life of the liver as much as possible. For example, the type and amount of protein that you consume needs to be carefully considered and restricted if you have advanced liver disease.

Meanwhile, somebody with fatty liver disease should be more mindful of their carbohydrate intake.

In this chapter, I provide the framework for a liver-friendly diet. However, it is important to keep in mind that everybody with liver disease is different. To establish a diet that is most optimal for *you*, be sure to talk with your doctor or dietitian/nutritionist. (If you do not have access to a dietitian or nutritionist, please be sure to check your health insurance plan to see what type of nutrition services, if any, may be covered. You may have to pay for a dietitian or nutritionist visit out-of-pocket.) In the following sections, I will touch on different aspects of liver-based nutrition.

■ Calories

Many studies suggest that the liver has specific "energy needs," and that when someone has liver disease, a significant energy deficit occurs in the liver. Understanding how many calories you need to take in is an important step in meeting the nutritional and energetic needs of the liver. The amount of calories you need depends on a variety of factors, including your weight, current health, and how advanced your illness is.

Generally, if you have cirrhosis, you will need to consume a slightly larger amount of calories than average. Some symptoms of cirrhosis, such as a loss of appetite, nausea, vomiting, abdominal pain, and anorexia, can make it difficult for someone with this condition to eat a balanced diet. Malnourishment often occurs in patients who have cirrhosis because the liver's ability to store and release energy is affected.

Consuming between 2,000 and 3,000 calories a day can provide the liver with the energy it needs to perform its functions adequately. These functions include building new cells and repairing itself. The specific caloric requirements depend on the patient's weight in kilograms. For example, if you weigh 70 kilograms (about 150 pounds), your total caloric requirements would be approximately 2,100 to 2,800 calories per day. (You need about 30 to 40 calories per kilogram of weight.) If you were in a hospitalized setting, your caloric goals would be on the higher end of this range.

Caloric requirements may differ depending on which condition you have. Studies researching caloric needs for non-alcoholic fatty liver disease (NAFLD) suggest opposite needs from those of cirrhosis. For example, a 2013 review compared patients who were fed a temporary high-calorie (hypercaloric) diet with patients who were fed a temporary low-calorie (hypocaloric) diet. The results found that those on the hyper-caloric diet had higher levels of a triglyceride that is often implicated in fatty liver disease. They also had a higher resistance to insulin. Those on the hypocaloric diet, however, rapidly showed improvements in their triglyceride levels. The review suggested that "ongoing excess caloric delivery directly contributes to the development of NAFLD."

A different study that researched the effects of diet in NAFLD recom-mended that, in terms of caloric intake, 40 to 50 percent of your total calo-ries come from foods that have a low glycemic index (i.e., foods that have decreased ability to raise blood glucose levels).

Talk with your doctor about what your individual calorie needs will be. Regardless of what your target number is, your calories should come from foods in a balanced and healthy diet, as I will discuss below.

◾ Carbohydrates, Fiber, and Sugar

Carbohydrates provide you with energy and are broken down into glu-cose. The recommended amount of carbohydrates for you to consume depends on your individual health. Diets either very high or severely restricted in carbohydrates can contribute to a worsening of liver disease.

On average, about 45 to 50 percent of your daily caloric intake should come from carbohydrates. Refer back to the example on page 137 of the indi-vidual who weighs 70 kilograms. If he needs at least 2,100 calories a day, then approximately 1,000 to 1,200 of those calories need to come from car-bohydrates. There are about four calories in every gram of carbohydrates, so this translates into about 250 to 300 grams of carbohydrates a day.

If you have fatty liver disease, or you have risk factors for it (such as metabolic syndrome), a diet more restricted in carbs is recommended. In these cases, carbohydrates should represent about 35 to 40 percent of your caloric intake. In the 70-kilogram person, this would equate to about 185 to 210 grams of carbohydrates a day. What you do not want to do is elim-inate carbs: Your body needs them to function.

Not only is the amount of carbohydrates you consume important, but the *type* of carbohydrates you consume is important, as well. You may have heard of simple carbohydrates (which are very quickly digested) and complex carbohydrates (which are high in dietary fiber). High levels of simple carbohydrates—also known as sugars—are associated with fatty liver disease. While the effects of fiber have not been studied as extensively, a study using rats found that a high-fiber diet can promote liver regeneration and reverse the effects of fatty liver disease.

A certain amount of carbohydrates are needed to balance out the amount of protein you take in each day. When there are not enough carbohydrates in the body to produce energy, the liver metabolizes protein for energy instead. This puts a larger strain on the liver because protein is more complicated to metabolize. Additionally, a lack of carbohydrates can cause your body to go into a state of *ketosis*. Ketosis is when the body relies on ketone bodies (a breakdown product from fats in the liver) for energy. If you have liver disease, ketosis can be a taxing and dangerous process on your liver.

Overall, a diet that is higher in complex carbohydrates and fiber and lower in simple sugars is recommended. Your liver depends on these carbohydrates to maintain energy and regulate the glucose in the blood.

■ Fat

A common characteristic in liver disease is trouble absorbing, storing, or digesting fat. Fatty liver disease, for example, is caused by fat buildup in the liver. Meanwhile, many cirrhosis patients' bodies are constantly breaking down fat—and once this fat has been used up, the body turns to breaking down muscle and tissue for energy instead.

The term "fat" often has a negative association, but some types of fats can be beneficial. Foods that contain monounsaturated or polyunsaturated fats (such as olive oil, avocados, nuts, and seeds) can have a protective effect in patients with NAFLD. In addition to consuming a diet lower in carbohydrates, increasing your consumption of monounsaturated and polyunsaturated fats is recommended by many studies, although further research is ongoing. For example, one study found that a diet rich in monounsaturated fats (such as the Mediterranean diet; see page 147) lowered levels of "bad" cholesterol, reduced blood pressure and glucose levels, and raised levels of "good" cholesterol in patients with fatty liver disease. Another study found that patients who took capsules of polyunsaturated fat showed significantly lower levels in their liver enzymes and cholesterol. Omega-3 fatty acids, primarily found in fish, are another beneficial type of polyunsaturated fat.

It is recommended that those with liver disease avoid trans fats completely and eat only a small amount of saturated fats. These fats are implicated not only in liver disease, but in cardiovascular disease as well. Trans fats are found almost exclusively in processed food (look for the word "hydrogenated" on the ingredients list). Studies using animals have found that replacing some low-fat foods in a diet with foods containing trans fats led to similar effects as a diet high in fat. Another study found that the saturated fats found in red meat were associated with a higher risk of chronic liver disease and liver cancer.

Try to keep total fat intake between 25 and 30 percent of your daily caloric intake. (In the example of 70-kilogram person, this would be about 60 to 90 grams of fat per day. One gram of fat is about nine calories.) Aim for most of this fat intake to be in the form of monounsaturated and polyunsaturated fats.

■ Potassium

Potassium is an electrolyte and mineral found in foods such as bananas, avocados, nuts, and potatoes. The amount of potassium you need depends on your nutritional status, certain prescription medication dosages, and how well your kidneys are functioning.

As you may recall from Chapter 5, spironolactone (brand name Aldactone) and furosemide (brand name Lasix) are frequently prescribed diuretics for the treatment of ascites and edema, respectively. Ascites and edema are common symptoms of liver disease. Remember that a potential side effect of spironolactone is hyperkalemia (high potassium levels). You may have already developed high potassium levels if your kidney function has been compromised. Patients who are taking furosemide (Lasix), meanwhile, may experience hypokalemia, or low potassium levels (this is a side effect of this medication). Your recommended daily intake of dietary potassium will depend a great deal on whether you are taking either of these medications and the severity of kidney disease, if it is present.

Your doctor will likely check your potassium and creatinine levels on routine blood work. If your potassium levels are low, she will likely recommend potassium in a prescription supplement, such as K-Dur.

■ Protein

Protein is important for rebuilding damaged liver cells. But if you have cirrhosis or advanced liver disease, you need to closely monitor your protein intake. The liver may not be able to efficiently process larger amounts of protein than you need because of cirrhosis. If you eat significantly more protein than the liver can handle, then you increase your risk of developing hepatic encephalopathy (the cognitive decline caused by the liver's inability to filter toxins from the bloodstream). This is because the liver produces ammonia, a toxic byproduct, whenever it breaks down protein. Normally, ammonia is eliminated from the body. But in the setting of advanced liver disease, the liver cannot properly dispose of ammonia, and it builds up in the bloodstream instead.

If possible, it is recommended that you try and fulfill your protein needs through vegetables and legumes instead of meat; meat produces higher ammonia levels than protein-rich vegetarian foods like beans, tofu, and Brussels sprouts. While maintaining a more vegetarian diet is not impossible, you often need to consume a larger variety of vegetarian protein sources to meet your daily protein needs.

When it comes to developing a nutrition plan, there is no one-size-fits-all approach. The degree of protein restriction depends both on your level of liver reserve and your existing nutritional status. Your doctor may set a target for you to consume a certain amount of protein based on your weight. Personally, I recommend between 1 to 1.2 grams of protein per kilogram of weight. So, in the case of the 70-kilogram patient, about 70 grams of protein a day would be recommended. If this patient is in the hospital, she may require a little more—about 80 to 84 grams of protein daily—to help speed recovery.

Many studies recommend that somebody who has hepatic encephalopathy—and is showing a high ammonia level—temporarily restrict her protein intake to 0.7 grams per kilogram. This is considered a moderate protein restriction. Once the patient has been treated, studies recommend increasing the daily protein intake back up to approximately 1 gram per kilogram of weight.

The important point is that severe protein restriction is not recommended, even in someone who has hepatic encephalopathy. Protein is still required for the body, especially in patients who experience muscle atrophy (weakness) as a result of advanced liver disease. Instead of severely limiting protein intake, the goal should be to prevent excess protein breakdown. This is especially true for patients who are already malnourished (as many with advanced liver disease are, because they do not have much of an appetite and can feel full very quickly). Everyone's nutritional needs and liver situations are different.

This section has gone over general guidelines regarding protein intake and the complications surrounding it that health professionals have to consider. *It is important to develop a personalized plan for protein intake with your doctor. The use of branched chain amino acids (discussed in the inset below) needs to be discussed with your physician first to determine if it is right for your own health situation.*

■ Sodium

Some sodium is good for you. Sodium can help balance the levels of electrolytes in your body, as well as the levels of fluid in your system. However, if you have liver disease, it is important to keep track of your sodium intake—especially if your symptoms include ascites, edema, dehydration, or high blood pressure. Excess sodium promotes fluid

Branched Chain Amino Acids' Benefit on Muscles

The use of *branched chain amino acids* (BCAA) can be helpful in reducing the rate of protein breakdown, which slows the buildup of toxins. The branched chain amino acids are *isoleucine, leucine,* and *valine.* They can be used to supplement the recommended protein intake.

Supplementing with BCAA is recommended for those who have cirrhosis. The levels of BCAA in patients who have cirrhosis can be much lower compared with those who have healthy livers. In one study, the use of BCAA delayed the onset of hepatic failure and improved the nutritional status of those with liver disease—for example, there were improvements in the levels of proteins such as albumin and prealbumin.

Liver disease—especially alcohol-induced cirrhosis—can affect muscle strength and muscle endurance. Over time, a type of muscle "disuse" atrophy (weakness) can develop. This is because the liver is not properly metabolizing protein; it is not using the protein to build and strengthen the muscles. Branched chain amino acids can reverse this muscle wasting and energy loss. The benefits of BCAA cannot be underestimated and their use should be strongly considered, especially if you are considering beginning an exercise program. (See Chapter 11 for more information about exercise programs and liver health.)

retention. Fluid retention and fluid backup puts additional pressure on your blood vessels.

According to the Food and Drug Administration, the recommended amount of sodium is 2,300 milligrams per day. If you have liver disease, it is recommended that you consume less than 1,500 milligrams of sodium a day. This degree of sodium restriction is especially recommended if you are experiencing significant ascites or edema; however, this limit can be difficult for many to adhere to.

Most fresh foods (such as fruits, vegetables, and unprocessed dairy products) are low in sodium. Although use of table salt in cooking and eating contributes only 5 to 10 percent to your daily sodium intake, it is best to avoid it. Using lemon juice, spices, or herbs on your food instead are tasty alternatives.

Avoid processed foods; the most common culprits of high sodium levels are frozen meals, soy sauce, canned soups and vegetables, deli meats, fast or fried food, and many snack foods that come in a bag, box, or can. If you are not sure, check the nutrition label. Anything that has above 460 milligrams per serving is considered a high-sodium food. In restaurants, ask for vegetables that are steamed, request dressings and sauces to be put on the side, avoid fried appetizers and meats (look for "baked," "broiled," and "grilled" instead), and ask if the kitchen can prepare your meal to fit your accommodations.

■ Vitamins and Minerals

Liver disease can cause malabsorption of nutrients. Even if you eat foods high in vitamins, the vitamins may not be processed in a way that benefits the rest of your body. Taking vitamin supplements can help get these important substances into your body, but talk with your doctor first. If you are unknowingly ingesting very high amounts of certain vitamins (such as vitamin A), it can further damage your liver instead of aid it.

Certain vitamins and minerals should be supplemented when you have liver disease. Key nutritional deficiencies in patients with a liver ailment include magnesium, selenium, thiamine, certain B vitamins, vitamin D, and zinc. Increasing your intake of these vitamins and minerals can improve morbidity and mortality (vitamin D), lessen the illness's severity (selenium), and significantly decrease the risk of developing certain neurologic complications, especially if they are caused by an alcohol-induced condition (thiamine).

However, some minerals do not need to be consumed in excess—even though they are included in many multivitamins. As you read about in Chapter 3, two hereditary conditions called hemochromatosis and Wilson's disease can damage the liver. Hemochromatosis is an excess of iron in the body, while Wilson's disease is an excess of copper. If you have hemochromatosis, avoid foods that are high in iron (such as red meat and shellfish) and multivitamins that are fortified with it. It is best not to cook with cast iron pots and pans. If you have Wilson's disease, avoid foods (such as chocolate, mushrooms, and some nuts), supplements, and cookware that contain copper.

FOODS AND DRINKS THAT CAN ENHANCE LIVER FUNCTION

The following is a short list of foods that are full of liver-friendly nutrients:

- **Avocado.** Avocados are rich in monounsaturated and polyunsaturated fats, which are important for the management of NAFLD. Avocados contain many other nutrients, including glutathione, the most important antioxidant for preserving liver health (see Chapter 10).

- **Coffee.** Several studies show that coffee may have a liver-protective effect, especially in patients with NAFLD. It is high in antioxidants. Coffee drinkers who have liver disease have reduced rates of developing cirrhosis. Note that the caffeine in coffee can aggravate certain symptoms, such as dehydration, ascites, and edema.

- **Fish.** Eating fish can reduce your risk of developing liver cancer. In a study regarding fish consumption and liver cancer, the authors demonstrated that eating one serving of fish a week can decrease your risk of developing this condition by as much as 18 percent. The authors suggested that the high concentration of polyunsaturated fat in fish is responsible for this protective effect.

- **Garlic and onion.** These two "superfoods" have been shown to possess detoxifying and liver-protective effects. A study in which rats with NAFLD were fed garlic and onion showed that the rats who ate these foods had a significant decrease in fatty liver and liver enzyme levels, compared with rats who did not eat garlic or onion. To get your daily "dose" of these, you can chop them up and add them to a salad or stir fry for a healthy, delicious meal.

- **Low-glycemic fruits.** Fruits that are low on the glycemic index, such as apples and berries, are very beneficial for those who have liver disease. These nutritious fruits contain carbohydrates but do not raise your blood glucose level too high.

- **Vegetables.** Any vegetable is a great source of fiber, vitamins, and vegetarian protein (as described on page 141), which can help decrease ammonia levels. Leafy green vegetables, such as kale or spinach, are especially beneficial.

- **White meat.** If you can't resist meat, choose white meat over red. In a study from the *Journal of the National Cancer Institute,* consumption of red meat was associated with a higher risk of developing liver cancer when compared with the consumption of white meat.

FOODS AND DRINKS TO AVOID

- **High-fructose corn syrup.** This is a highly unhealthy sweetener. Many foods have high-fructose corn syrup added to them; it is important to check the ingredients list on nutrition labels. When fructose is consumed, it travels straight to your liver. As it can only be processed by the liver, it is found in much higher levels in the liver than in other organs. However, fructose is very difficult for the liver to metabolize. High fructose levels increase the amount of fat that is formed in the liver; this dramatically increases the risk of developing a condition such as NAFLD or NASH.

- **Red meat.** Red meat is high in saturated fat, which can worsen fatty liver disease. It is also very high in protein and can cause more ammonia production than vegetarian protein sources, so it is not the best choice if you are at risk of developing hepatic encephalopathy.

- **Soft and sugar-sweetened drinks.** In a study from the *Canadian Journal of Gastroenterology,* the dietary habits of individuals with fatty liver disease were evaluated over a three-year period. It was noted that over 80 percent of them consumed sugar-sweetened soft drinks on a daily basis. Decreasing or eliminating sugar-sweetened soft drinks is only beneficial for your liver, as well as for your overall health.

A REVIEW OF COMMON DIETS

Some well-established, popular diets place an emphasis on foods that are good for the liver. Since these diets often have books, websites, and large followings devoted to them, it can be easier to follow them than it is to create a nutrition plan on your own. This section will review some popular diets that I feel can be beneficial for liver health.

■ DASH Diet

The DASH (Dietary Approaches to Stop Hypertension) diet is a nutrition plan that has been recommended and proven to be beneficial for individuals with hypertension (high blood pressure). It also has many helpful effects and improves morbidity and mortality in individuals with congestive heart failure (CHF). The DASH diet is plant-based, with daily recommended servings of fruits and vegetables in addition to whole grains.

This diet has positive effects for individuals with liver disease. In one study, about sixty patients diagnosed with NAFLD were randomized and followed for approximately two months. One group was instructed to follow a DASH diet-based nutrition plan (by consuming high servings of fruits, vegetables, and whole grains), while the other group served as the control group. Both groups adopted a calorie-restricted diet and consumed similar amounts of carbohydrates, fats, and protein; the difference was in the selection of food choices.

The authors noted that the individuals who adopted the DASH-associated diet plan lost more weight and lowered both their liver enzyme levels and triglyceride levels. The researchers concluded that the type of foods consumed by the DASH diet group accounted for the significant difference between the two groups.

■ Gluten-Free Diet

Celiac disease, a condition in which patients cannot digest gluten in food, is managed through a gluten-free diet. Note that it can potentially cause cirrhosis; celiac disease may account for 2 percent of all causes of cirrhosis. The reverse of this is also true: The number of individuals with cirrhosis who also have been diagnosed with celiac disease is about twice that of the general population. Because these two conditions can occur together, it may be wise for you to be evaluated for celiac disease. However, this is not a current standard of care.

Studies have shown that adhering to a gluten-free diet can improve liver enzyme tests in those who have cirrhosis. One study followed four people who had both advanced liver disease and celiac disease. These patients adopted a gluten-free diet, and within months, all four showed healthier results in their liver function tests. Their symptoms vastly improved while on the diet. Although the study tested a small sample size, it suggests that following a gluten-free diet can significantly help those who have both celiac disease and liver disease.

Even if you do not have celiac disease, following a gluten-free diet may improve your symptoms of liver disease. Another piece of good news is that it is becoming easier to follow a gluten-free diet. In recent years, the number of gluten-free products available in grocery stores and restaurants has increased, allowing those who follow this diet to buy celiac-friendly versions of bread, pasta, and more.

Naturally gluten-free foods include unprocessed beans, seeds, and nuts; eggs; fish (without marinades or breading); fruits and vegetables; and most dairy products. Contrary to popular belief, many grains can also be a part of a gluten-free diet, such as buckwheat, flax, rice, soy, and quinoa.

Foods to avoid—unless they are specifically labeled "gluten-free"—include beer; bread; cereal; chips; crackers; imitation meat or seafood; pasta; pastries; and sauces, such as salad dressing, soy sauce, and gravy. If you are in doubt about a certain product, read the ingredients list. Avoid items that include barley, durum flour, rye, semolina, spelt, and wheat flour. Foods that are labeled "wheat-free" may still contain gluten. If you are not sure if a food contains gluten, contact the manufacturer or check with your doctor or dietitian.

Keep in mind that "gluten-free" does not always equate to "healthy"—so, as with any diet for liver disease, place an emphasis on fruits and vegetables and avoid foods high in sugar and cholesterol.

■ Mediterranean Diet

If you have a fatty liver or have risk factors for the development of NAFLD, then adopting the Mediterranean diet may be beneficial.

The Mediterranean diet places a focus not only on fruits and vegetables, but also on nuts, grains, and healthy fats and oils. Olive oil is a mainstay of this diet. The Mediterranean diet also focuses on reducing the consumption of processed meats. Red wine is often included in a

The Mediterranean Diet and Red Wine

A low-to-moderate amount of red wine is often recommended in a Mediterranean diet. However, as you learned in Chapter 3, even that "one glass of wine at night" can aggravate the liver. When you have liver disease, you want to avoid alcohol consumption. You can still follow a Mediterranean diet without this addition. Resveratrol, an antioxidant, is thought to be the main beneficial component of red wine. Taking resveratrol supplements can give you the benefits of red wine without experiencing the damaging effects of alcohol.

Mediterranean diet, but as you have learned, total avoidance of alcohol is necessary to the treatment of liver disease (see inset "The Mediterranean Diet and Red Wine" above).

A 2014 study defined the Mediterranean diet as "a collection of eating habits. . . . characterized by a high consumption of fruit, vegetables, legumes, and complex carbohydrates, with a moderate consumption of fish and the use of olive oil as the main source of fats." This study and several others have demonstrated this is a very liver-friendly diet, especially if NAFLD is present. This diet can decrease insulin resistance and the levels of the liver enzymes. This is mainly due to the monounsaturated and polyunsaturated fats (see page 139) that are present in olive oil and in many other foods included in the Mediterranean diet.

The Mediterranean diet also has been shown to improve cardiovascular health, reduce blood glucose levels (helpful for patients who have diabetes), and stave off weight gain. These conditions can often precede or co-occur with liver disease. One of the easiest parts of following this diet is that it is not a traditional diet plan, per se. Instead of restricting foods, it is a framework that emphasizes using oils and unsaturated fats to change your eating habits for the better.

SUMMARY

A healthy nutrition plan plays a significant role not only in the prevention of liver disease, but also its treatment. Since the food and drinks you consume are processed and metabolized in the liver, it is important to be mindful of what you are eating. Everyone with liver disease has different needs, but in general, it is best to maintain a diet that emphasizes fruits, vegetables, and whole grains. Diets should promote monounsaturated and polyunsaturated fats, while avoiding saturated and trans fats and foods high in cholesterol, sodium, and sugar. In advanced liver disease, pay particular attention to protein consumption.

Whichever nutrition plan you decide to follow should provide a framework, but at the same time not be so restrictive that it is too difficult to maintain long-term. Studies show that the DASH diet, the gluten-free diet, and the Mediterranean diet are among the popular diets that have significant liver-protective benefits. The development of a personalized nutrition plan that specifically works for you needs to be discussed with your doctor.

10

Using Natural Supplements and Herbs for Liver Disease

As you have learned, the liver is responsible for processing the nutrients you consume and releasing them into the bloodstream to be transported to other parts of the body. However, when you have liver disease, this ability of the liver is compromised. Even if you eat a healthy and balanced diet, the nutrients from those foods may not be adequately processed in the liver. Many people turn to supplements and herbs for a few reasons. For one, they can be a way to help correct any underlying nutritional deficiencies that may be present. Another reason is to maintain or even help improve liver function.

Supplements are antioxidants, extracts, herbs, minerals, or vitamins that come in pill, capsule, powder, or liquid forms. By definition, a supplement is something that is "added on" to enhance the user's health. They are considered to be "natural" alternatives to Western medicines, and you do not need a prescription to use or buy them. However, just because something is natural does not always mean it is good for you. Just like some prescription and over-the-counter medicines, some supplements can damage your liver if they are taken in large amounts or in combination with other treatments.

However, many supplements and herbs can be used to help improve and maintain your liver health. More often than not, these will be recommended or given to you by natural-based health practitioners. In this chapter, you will read about the most common supplements that can support liver health. As you will read, these supplements have benefits above and beyond their ability to protect the liver. Many protect other organs in your body, and some can be used in the treatment of other conditions.

It is important to keep in mind that some supplements may not be right for you, depending on existing health conditions. Everybody's system is different and not everybody will process a supplement in the same way. Always check with your health care provider(s) before you begin taking a supplement. Your physician will be able to confirm whether the supplement will interact well with or interfere with any other medications you are taking.

HOW SUPPLEMENTS ARE PREPARED AND ADMINISTERED

When you have liver disease, you need to be more attentive than ever to what you consume and put into your body. Your liver is in a sensitive state and too much of a harmful substance can damage it further. However, many of the supplements described in this chapter can protect it and give it the "boost" it needs to function more effectively.

When you shop for supplements, keep in mind that they are not thoroughly regulated by the Food and Drug Administration (FDA) the way prescription medications are. In other words, prescription medicine has been clinically tested, has been proven to be effective, and must have all of the active and inactive ingredients listed on the label. Supplements and herbs are not subject to this regulation. They are considered "safe until proven unsafe." The majority of supplements on the market are, indeed, safe to consume. However, the lack of regulation also leaves room for dishonest companies to add in heavy metals or pesticides. Some products may contain additional ingredients that are not noted on the label (or they may lack the main ingredient they claim to have!). Weight loss and bodybuilding supplements tend to be the most frequent offenders of deceitful marketing. Trust your intuition and be wary of manufacturers that do not have contact information, or that make outrageous claims without any evidence—supplements are not legally allowed to claim that they can diagnose, treat, or cure a disease.

With that being said, there are many supplemental products that can help maintain your liver health, make you feel more energized, and can help relieve some of your symptoms. Some products can even counteract damage from acetaminophen overdose; others may contribute to lower liver enzyme levels. Categories of supplements include antioxidants; herbs and botanicals; vitamins and minerals; and specialty supplements (e.g., caffeine and probiotics). Having a balanced level of each of these components in your body is essential for good health. In the sections below, I will discuss the benefits of the top supplements in each category.

Keep in mind that this chapter is meant to be a general guide to these herbs and supplements. It is not meant to be a replacement for treatment by a doctor. Always speak with your health care providers before beginning a supplement program.

ANTIOXIDANTS

Antioxidants are substances that protect the cells from the effects of free radicals (highly reactive, unstable molecules). Having too many free radicals in the body has been linked to illnesses such as heart disease and cancer. When there is an imbalance between antioxidants and free radicals, it is called *oxidative stress*. Antioxidants neutralize the damage that can occur from free radicals or oxidative stress.

Many people who have liver disease are also found to be undergoing oxidative stress, so it makes sense that antioxidants have been shown in several studies to help liver damage. Antioxidants can also help by speeding up the process of cell detoxification.

The antioxidants that have been studied most in relation to the liver are alpha lipoic acid, glutathione, melatonin, and N-acetylcysteine. In addition to these, many vitamins and minerals—such as vitamin C and vitamin E—are considered antioxidants as well. (See the section "Vitamins and Minerals" on page 159.)

■ Alpha Lipoic Acid

Alpha lipoic acid (*lip-oh-ick*), or ALA, is a supplement that has antioxidant properties. It has been demonstrated in animal-based studies to reduce the degree of damage caused by oxidative stress. The body produces ALA on its own, but levels can decrease if liver disease is present. ALA has many important functions, including energy production in the cells, detoxification, and brain wellness. It can increase the levels of the "master antioxidant," glutathione, in the cells (see "Glutathione" on page 154).

ALA has also been studied in the treatment of diabetes and metabolic syndrome (a group of risk factors or conditions that are associated with serious illnesses, such as heart disease). It has been found to be effective in decreasing the cells' resistance to insulin. Because of the strong connection between diabetes, metabolic syndrome, and the development of a fatty liver, this supplement is highly recommended if you have NAFLD, although it can protect against other causes of liver ailments as well.

Alpha lipoic acid can be given both orally and intravenously. The usual dose that I tend to start with is 200 milligrams daily; I then increase the dose by 200 milligrams each week, up to a maximum dosage of 600 to 800 milligrams a day (taken in two divided doses).

It is important to note that there is a reason why you need to be careful and increase the dose slowly when you begin taking this supplement: This minimizes the risk of developing a low blood sugar level (also referred to as hypoglycemia). Because this supplement decreases insulin resistance, it increases the risk of developing hypoglycemia, especially at higher doses. You may recall that one of the liver's functions is to increase glucose levels in the blood when it needs to (e.g., when the body is stressed or if the blood glucose level is too low). In cases of advanced liver disease, the liver may not be functioning well enough to regulate the glucose level; consequently, hypoglycemia can occur. If your blood glucose levels are in the lower range (for example, less than 70 milligrams per deciliter) on a consistent basis, then you may be able to tolerate only low doses of ALA, if at all. If I start a patient on this supplement, I will ask him to have blood work done more than once to measure his blood glucose level over time.

Alpha lipoic acid can be purchased as an oral supplement in natural products and health food stores, but as always, check with your physician before you begin to take it (especially if you have a low blood sugar level or are at risk for hypoglycemia).

■ Glutathione

Glutathione (gloot-uh-thigh-own) is one of the most important and powerful cell antioxidants. Like alpha lipoic acid, it is naturally produced by the body, but its levels can become depleted when the body is undergoing stress or disease. It is mainly produced and stored in the liver and is transported through bile. Glutathione's roles include reducing oxidative stress in liver cells, protecting against free radical damage, and maintaining the viability of the cells. It is sometimes called the "master antioxidant" because it has important detoxifying and metabolizing functions in nearly every system in the body. It can also regulate and recycle other antioxidants. Some of the supplements that you read about in this chapter not only have antioxidant and anti-inflammatory properties of their own, but they also increase glutathione levels in the cells.

Glutathione has been implicated in the treatment of dozens of conditions, ranging from eye conditions like glaucoma to blood conditions such as anemia to, of course, liver disease. If you have liver cancer, glutathione has also been shown to counteract some painful side effects of chemotherapy. Glutathione helps rebuild body tissue and maintain the immune system. Its importance in your overall health cannot be underestimated.

As you may have guessed, cells that are very low in glutathione are more at risk of developing injury over time. Glutathione depletion can increase the risk of cell death. As you read about in Chapter 5, high doses of acetaminophen (Tylenol) can be one cause of severe glutathione depletion. Poor diet, high exposure to toxins, and stress can also decrease glutathione levels. One of the basic tenets of protecting your liver health is to look for ways to replenish glutathione and boost levels of it in the cells.

Glutathione can be taken orally, but it needs to be consumed along with the amino acid *cysteine* to help it get into the cells. I myself take a supplement once or twice a day that contains a combination of glutathione and cysteine, as well as vitamin C. Glutathione can also be given intravenously by a health care provider to protect against blood and kidney issues, to treat diabetes, or to protect against the side effects of chemotherapy. Additionally, it is naturally found in many foods, especially green vegetables such as asparagus and spinach.

◼ Melatonin

Melatonin (mel-uh-tone-in) is a hormonal supplement that is often used as a sleep aid. However, several studies have found it to have strong antioxidant properties, as well, which suggests that it can benefit patients with liver disease. The research demonstrates that melatonin may be especially beneficial as a potential therapy for NAFLD.

One study using rats with acute and chronic liver disease found that rats who were treated with melatonin had significantly improved results on their liver enzyme tests than rats in a control group who were treated with a placebo. The rats who were treated with melatonin also had a more normal ratio of liver weight to body weight. The melatonin-treated rats had lower levels of oxidative stress molecules, showing that melatonin may have free radical-scavenging properties similar to those of ALA and glutathione. The study concluded that melatonin treatment may be an effective method to reduce liver injury that has been caused by oxidative stress.

In a lab-based study, when melatonin was given to mice that had NAFLD, the melatonin supplementation was found to reverse some of the fat deposition and improve glucose handling in the mice livers. In another, population-based study, forty-two patients with non-alcoholic steatohepatitis (NASH) were given either 5 milligrams of melatonin twice a day or a placebo. The patients were followed over a period of twelve weeks. Patients who were given melatonin showed substantial reduction in liver enzymes, including alanine transaminase (ALT), aspartate transaminase (AST), and gamma-glutamyl transferase (GGT), compared with patients who took the placebo. Both of these studies demonstrate melatonin's positive effect in patients with fatty liver. While the optimal dose and duration of melatonin for this condition is still being researched, it seems reasonable to consider adding a melatonin supplement to your daily regimen.

Melatonin is sold over-the-counter as an oral supplement in most drugstores and natural products stores. It has not been discovered to have serious side effects in most people, but check with your health care provider before taking it, especially if you are already on other medications that may cause drowsiness. The usual dosage is around 3 to 5 milligrams a day to start.

■ N-Acetylcysteine

N-acetylcysteine (NAC) is one of the cornerstones of holistic liver health management. It is a potent antioxidant that helps to raise levels of glutathione in the cells. In fact, NAC is such a powerful liver antioxidant that it is often used by transplant centers to help maintain the viability of a new liver in patients who undergo a transplant.

NAC is derived from an amino acid called cysteine, which is needed to synthesize glutathione. By replenishing the cysteine, NAC boosts glutathione levels. Just like the other antioxidants described in this section, NAC is an active scavenger of free radicals and has been found to reduce the negative effects of oxidative stress. A study comparing NAC to vitamin C in the treatment of NAFLD found that the patients who were treated with NAC had a more significant decrease in their liver enzymes.

This supplement can be consumed either orally or intravenously, depending on what it is treating. For example, it is often taken orally for detoxification and liver-protective purposes. It is given intravenously for conditions such as acetaminophen overdose and hepatorenal syndrome (kidney failure that is caused by liver disease), usually in the hospital setting. NAC has been shown to be very effective in treating patients who

Signs of an Acetaminophen Overdose

As mentioned in Chapter 5, Tylenol is not the only medication that contains acetaminophen. Many medications that treat colds and the flu (such as DayQuil/NyQuil or Sudafed) or that manage pain (such as Percocet or Vicodin) contain some amount of acetaminophen. Many people unknowingly ingest a larger amount of this drug than they need or than their bodies can handle. Over time, this can severely injure the liver. Acetaminophen overdose is one of the most common causes of poisoning in the world. Signs of an overdose include:

- Abdominal pain
- Coma
- Diarrhea
- Jaundice
- Nausea or upset stomach
- Seizure
- Sweating
- Vomiting

To protect your liver, consult with your doctor about the medications you are taking and make sure that the amount of acetaminophen in them (if any) is a safe amount for you. Call poison control immediately if you believe you have overdosed.

suffer an acetaminophen overdose. The damage from an overdose is minimized because of the NAC's ability to replenish glutathione levels in the liver, which allows for the liver to metabolize and eliminate the acetaminophen without toxic side effects. NAC can be a vital way to prevent severe liver injury or liver failure following an acetaminophen overdose (see "Signs of an Acetaminophen Overdose" inset above).

The most common oral dose of NAC is 600 milligrams taken twice a day, although this dose can go up to 1,200 milligrams twice a day. The dosage can vary and is usually based on a person's weight.

HERBS

Before modern medication was invented, herbs and plants were widely used to treat wounds and diseases. Today, they are still in popular use as supplements for their natural healing qualities. Two herbs that are most commonly used to treat liver disease are milk thistle and turmeric.

▓ Milk Thistle

Milk thistle is an herb found throughout the world that has been used for thousands of years to treat liver disease. It is one of the best and more extensively studied supplements for this purpose. Milk thistle is also known as silymarin, which is its main ingredient; silymarin has anti-inflammatory properties. There are numerous ways in which this potent herb exerts its protective effects.

Milk thistle is an antioxidant; it can help protect the hepatocyte cells from oxidative stress and free radical formation. Some studies suggest that milk thistle may preserve liver function by binding to the toxins and preventing them from entering the liver cells. In addition, some animal-based studies suggest that it can decrease the degree of toxin-induced damage. Other studies have demonstrated that milk thistle may also help in the treatment of hepatitis (including viral hepatitis and alcoholic hepatitis). The silymarin in milk thistle has been shown to strengthen the walls of the cell to prevent toxins from entering; provoke toxin-fighting enzymes to protect the body; and block disease-causing free radicals.

In addition to helping treat liver disease, some research has suggested that milk thistle can be used in the treatment of diabetes and high cholesterol. Milk thistle has been shown to lower blood sugar levels, insulin resistance, and levels of "bad" LDL cholesterol. Diabetes, high cholesterol, and liver disease often all go hand-in-hand; this information supports the idea that milk thistle can help those with liver illnesses who also have pre-existing diabetes.

I tend to recommend a capsule form to my patients, starting at 100 milligrams taken twice a day. This can be increased slowly to anywhere from 200 to 600 milligrams daily. Milk thistle rarely causes side effects, although it should be avoided if you have a ragweed allergy. It should also not be taken by pregnant or breastfeeding women, or women who have certain hormonal disorders (as milk thistle may take on some of the effects of a hormone called estrogen).

▓ Turmeric

Turmeric is an herb with anti-inflammatory properties that is also an effective antioxidant. Its main component is curcumin, whose benefits in a number of diseases are being studied. Turmeric is often used as a spice in food or as a food dye, but it is also sold as a supplement. Studies have demonstrated that turmeric has liver-protective effects. For example, an animal-based study demonstrated that the curcumin in turmeric could successfully treat jaundice and reduce the formation of gallstones. It also reduced the amount of fibrosis (scarring) in the liver.

Turmeric may be especially beneficial for those with viral hepatitis. The peer-reviewed journal *Gut* reviewed a lab-based study concerning the effects of turmeric on virus-induced liver disease. The authors noted that not only did turmeric help prevent the virus from entering the cell, it also helped to prevent further transmission of the virus from one cell to another. This herb seems to have the ability to prevent a virus from penetrating the cells and spreading throughout the body—that is such amazing physiology!

Additional protective effects of turmeric were noted in an animal model; those fed turmeric were noted to have lower cholesterol levels and were less likely to develop a fatty liver compared with a control group.

Turmeric can be consumed in a number of ways, including a spice that you can incorporate into your food. For simplicity's sake, I suggest a capsule form. I tend to start at doses of 400 milligrams daily, which can increase to 800 milligrams a day, taken with food. The highest dose I recommend is 1,500 milligrams, taken in divided doses throughout the day.

Please be aware that turmeric does have blood thinning properties; if you are taking other prescription blood thinners, then you need to consult with your doctor or health care practitioner before consuming turmeric.

If you have gallbladder problems, then you also need to consult with your doctor before taking turmeric. Turmeric can increase bile flow through the gallbladder, which can worsen an acute gallbladder attack.

VITAMINS AND MINERALS

Vitamins and minerals are found in nearly every food, either naturally or artificially added. Everyone needs to consume a certain amount of vitamins and minerals every day, although too much of some vitamins can be harmful (see inset "How Much is Too Much?" on page 161). Below, I explain the benefits of selenium and vitamin D in particular when treating your liver.

■ Selenium

Selenium is a mineral that is found naturally in foods such as nuts, seeds, seafood, and grains. It is important for maintaining a healthy immune system and for preserving the integrity and viability of the cells. Several studies suggest that this mineral may be especially helpful in promoting liver health and fighting liver disease, especially viral hepatitis. An article from the *Saudi Journal of Gastroenterology* evaluated subjects in Pakistan, where the rates of hepatitis B and C are endemic. They noted that the patients with hepatitis B or C had lower levels of selenium in their bodies than healthy individuals had. It was suggested that selenium deficiency may play a role in the progression of viral hepatitis. Another study demonstrated that drug users infected with hepatitis C and/or the human immunodeficiency virus (HIV) showed lower levels of selenium.

Given the results of the above studies, an important clinical question becomes: Does selenium supplementation decrease a patient's viral load (the quantity of a virus measured in the blood)? The results are somewhat mixed. In a study from the *Archives of Internal Medicine,* investigators noted that patients diagnosed with HIV who were taking 200 micrograms of selenium a day experienced a reduction in the HIV viral load.

What about viral hepatitis? In one study, selenium (as well as vitamin C and vitamin E) was given to patients with chronic hepatitis C. While the patients did experience an increase in antioxidant load, neither the patients' liver enzymes nor their viral burdens decreased. Further research is ongoing; this study shows that while selenium may help decrease oxidative stress in the liver, it may not be beneficial in reducing liver enzymes.

Selenium is a trace mineral, meaning that it is needed only in small amounts (around 55 micrograms a day). Generally, a regular, healthy diet is an adequate source of selenium. However, if you and your doctor have agreed that a selenium supplement will benefit you, note that the safe upper limit for adults is 400 micrograms a day.

■ Vitamin D

Vitamin D is one of the most important vitamins; it is responsible for regulating and metabolizing calcium in the body, and it has been suggested that it may prevent conditions such as cancer and diabetes. It is attained naturally from sunlight, and is added to many foods (such as milk).

How is vitamin D related to liver health? Well, an interesting study from the journal *Endocrine* reviewed the lab data of over 2,500 individuals. The researchers noted an inverse relationship between vitamin D levels and liver disease incidence—that is, higher levels of vitamin D were asso-

How Much is Too Much?

Taking or consuming the recommended amount of vitamins and minerals is important to your health. To enhance your wellbeing, it may be appealing to take a broad multivitamin that is comprised of high doses of numerous vitamins and minerals. However, as the saying goes, sometimes too much of a good thing can be bad for you. In high amounts, certain vitamins and minerals can actually cause more problems in your liver than they solve. These are the most prominent vitamins that can be harmful in high doses:

- **Vitamin A.** Vitamin A contributes to normal vision, the immune system, and to the health of your most important organs. Vitamin A in the beta-carotene form is considered safe and nontoxic. However, some other forms of vitamin A can accumulate in your liver (where it is stored) and cause joint and bone pain, headaches, nausea, skin irritation, and in severe cases, coma. The recommended upper intake level of vitamin A is 3,300 micrograms per day for adults.

- **Vitamin E.** In the recommended amount (15 milligrams per day), vitamin E is a great antioxidant that protects your body from free radicals. It also is important in preserving your immune system and preventing vessel-clogging blood clots. However, consuming more than 1,000 mg of vitamin E per day in supplement form can cause excessive internal or external bleeding. It can also interact with blood thinning medications or chemotherapy.

- **Iron.** As you have learned, iron is stored in the liver. Iron is an important component for producing the red blood cells that carry oxygen throughout your body. However, having too much iron in your system (e.g., if you have hemochromatosis) can put a lot of stress on your liver. The recommended daily amount of iron is about 8 milligrams for men and 18 milligrams for women, although this amount may be higher if you are a vegetarian or pregnant. The recommended upper limit is 45 milligrams per day. If you have liver disease or are at risk of developing one, it is best to avoid multivitamins that have iron added to them. Many brands carry iron-free versions of their multivitamins.

ciated with a lower number of people being diagnosed with liver disease, and vice versa. Another study demonstrated that those who were diagnosed with NAFLD in particular had lower levels of this important vitamin. Since vitamin D is a fat-soluble vitamin, having a malfunctioning liver may prevent it from being adequately absorbed (due to the liver's decreased ability to metabolize fat). This could lead to a deficiency.

One of the aforementioned studies found that lower vitamin D levels were correlated with high levels of liver enzymes, but the exact connection between vitamin D and liver enzymes continues to be researched. However, if you have been diagnosed with liver disease or you have the risk factors, you should consider having your level of vitamin D measured. For most people, the goal is to have a level between 40 and 50 picograms per milliliter. I tend to start patients at a minimum dose of 2,000 IU (international units) per day, adjusting the dose in accordance with any change in their levels.

OTHER SUPPLEMENTS

Coffee and probiotics, the two supplements listed below, do not entirely fall under the categories of antioxidant, herbs, or vitamins, although they do share some benefits with these other supplements. Both coffee and probiotics have been shown in various studies to improve symptoms of various liver diseases.

■ Coffee

Coffee, one of the world's favorite beverages, has been demonstrated to have protective effects against many liver diseases. While caffeine is the most notable ingredient in coffee, it is difficult to pinpoint whether it is the caffeine or another compound that is responsible for coffee's beneficial effects on the liver.

A 2014 report from the *Journal of Gastroenterology and Hepatology* analyzed over a dozen studies that researched the relationship between coffee and liver disease. The studies were in agreement that higher coffee intake was associated with lower risk of fatty liver, non-alcoholic steatohepatitis, and even hepatocellular carcinoma (HCC), a form of liver cancer. The relationship between increased coffee intake and decreased HCC risk is very consistent across multiple studies. In one, it was determined that drinking more than four cups of coffee a week cut the risk of developing HCC in half in those who already had chronic hepatitis B. Another meta-analysis studied coffee's effect on cirrhosis in over 400,000 people and found that having an extra two cups of coffee per day may reduce the risk of cirrhosis by 44 percent.

It is also worth noting that coffee has antioxidant qualities. As you learned on page 153, antioxidants protect the body from oxidative stress and free radicals. One trial compared participants who consumed 800 milliliters (a little over three cups) of coffee every day for five days with participants who only drank water. The researchers found that oxidative damage to DNA was decreased by 12 percent in those who drank coffee. Although it is too early to start calling coffee a miracle cure for your liver, the evidence points to it being an addition to your diet that can work in your favor.

■ Probiotics

Probiotics are "good" bacteria that keep your digestive system and intestines healthy. But probiotics do not just have beneficial effects on the intestines; they are also beneficial for the liver. I mentioned in Chapter 1 that one of the functions of the liver is to help the digestive system process nutrients and metabolize fat, carbohydrates, and protein. Consuming probiotics enhances the good bacteria's ability to help the liver carry out these functions. There are many different probiotic products available; see the inset "A Guide to Probiotics" on pages 164 to 165 for information about the various aspects of these supplements.

The ability of the liver to process a dietary load—especially one that is higher in protein—can be compromised, depending on the severity of the liver disease. Liver disease can cause changes in the types and amount of bacteria that are present in the gut; for example, one report found that in cirrhosis patients, there was a reduction in *Bifidobacterium* (a beneficial bacteria) and increases in *Enterobacteriaceae* and *Enterococcus* (infection-causing bacteria). Some evidence points to the ability of probiotics to bind to and immobilize liver-damaging toxins and carcinogens in the gut.

Probiotics may be helpful for treating hepatic encephalopathy. As you may recall, this condition is a complication of advanced liver disease. It is caused by the buildup of ammonia, a toxic byproduct that the liver becomes unable to process and clear. Probiotics can help by protecting the intestines from the damaging effects of ammonia. They can be used in conjunction with prescription medications (described in Chapter 5) to

A Guide to Probiotics

There are so many different types and brands of probiotics out there. How do you know if you have an effective one? There are certain characteristics that you want to be sure to examine when you are purchasing a probiotic:

- **Quantity.** How many colony forming units of bacteria does your probiotic contain? A "decent" probiotic will contain approximately 3 to 5 billion colony forming units per tablet or capsule.

- **Strains.** What are the different types of organisms in your probiotic? Not all probiotics contain the same organisms. You want a probiotic that has several species of *Lactobacillus* and *Bifidobacterium*. These strains can reduce inflammation and maintain homeostasis (acid/alkaline balance) in the intestines. You may want to look for a probiotic that also has *Saccharomyces boulardii*, which can have a protective effect on the intestines.

- **Directions.** When taking the probiotic, be sure to read the directions for dosage and storage information. Some probiotics need to be refrigerated, some don't. Probiotics in capsule form that can be stored at room temperature are the easiest to maintain. Begin with one capsule a day. Many probiotics are taken on an empty stomach at least thirty minutes prior to taking other prescription medications and supplements, as

help manage hepatic encephalopathy. Probiotics may also help delay the development of this condition. Note that in the studies, there did not seem to be a reduction in ammonia levels, but clarity, thinking, and cognition still improved in patients.

Some strains of probiotics have anti-inflammatory properties in the intestines, which is why they are often recommended for treating diseases in the intestines and bowel. In addition to having these significant anti-inflammatory properties, think of probiotics as "helping to give the liver a breather," or easing the workload of the liver, since they help the liver carry out its roles in digestion (see inset "Should Probiotics Be Given in the Hospital Setting?" on page 166).

Probiotics have been studied in various types of liver disease. A meta-analysis done in the *Annals of Hepatology* journal in 2014 looked at several randomized, controlled trials concerning the effect of probiotics in patients with non-alcoholic fatty liver disease. (Abnormal intestinal flora to allow for maximum absorption of the probiotic. However, double-check the directions on your probiotics; different brands may have different instructions.

- **Possible interactions.** Because antibiotic medications can kill off both good and bad bacteria in your body, you may want to use a probiotic to balance out the effects of an antibiotic. However, if you are taking an antibiotic, don't take it at the same time of day as a probiotic: Doing so will "kill off" the bacterial flora of the probiotic and minimize its effectiveness. Instead, it is better to take the antibiotic first thing in the morning and then take the probiotic several hours later (preferably in the late afternoon or early evening).

  Be aware that many supplements and herbs have natural "antibiotic-like" properties. Because of this, they can have a similar effect to taking a prescribed antibiotic. Examples of these include garlic, Echinacea, oil of oregano, olive leaf extract, and resveratrol. Take probiotics at a different time of day from these supplements.

  Probiotics are generally very safe, but some strains may interact with antifungal or immunosuppressant medications. Consult with your doctor first if you are on any of these medications and are interested in taking probiotics.

and increased inflammation are thought to be contributing factors in the development of NAFLD.) In more than two-thirds of the trials reviewed, the study subjects who received a probiotic showed a reduction in their liver enzyme tests.

SUPPLEMENTS TO AVOID

Just because something is natural does not always mean that it is good for you. The herbs listed in this section can have detrimental effects on your liver and should be avoided.

■ Comfrey

Comfrey is an herb that has been used topically (on the skin) for treating wounds and inflammation. However, consuming comfrey orally has been linked to cases of acute liver disease and injury. This is because comfrey

Should Probiotics Be Given in a Hospital Setting?

When a person with advanced liver disease is admitted to the hospital, it is usually because of a complication, such as hepatic encephalopathy or a sudden and acute illness. The acute illness (for example, pneumonia) may not seem related to the liver function, but regardless, any sudden sickness can be stressful on the liver. The liver is likely not up to task of combating the additional strain; it does not have the reserve. I think that the use of probiotics can really help in this regard. This is a topic of debate among health care professionals, but I am of the opinion that probiotics can help in a hospital setting by decreasing the workload and burden on the liver.

contains substances called *pyrrolizidine alkaloids,* which (when metabolized) are converted into products that are toxic to the liver. Its internal use has been banned in the United States.

■ Kava Kava

Kava kava is an herbal remedy that is typically used in tea or capsule form to treat anxiety. While evidence points to kava being an effective treatment for anxiety, there is concern that it can cause severe liver damage and even liver failure. Its use has been banned in Poland and is regulated in several other countries. There have been case studies in which patients who used kava developed liver disease to the point of needing a liver transplant. However, it has not been determined whether kava itself caused the liver damage in these situations, or if the kava products were contaminated with mold or other outside substances.

■ Weight Loss Supplements

There are many supplements on the market that claim to be natural, effective, and easy methods to lose weight, burn fat, and build muscle. However, many of these products are unsafe to consume, especially if you have liver disease. As with other natural supplements, weight loss supplements are not regulated by the Food and Drug Administration. Companies do not need their marketing to be approved by the FDA before the products are released. However, the FDA can remove a product from shelves after complaints against it have been received and verified. Many of these products can be tainted with hidden ingredients; some have even been found to contain prescription drugs. If you are considering using a weight loss supplement, check with your doctor first to make sure it is a legitimate, safe product.

SUMMARY

In your journey to restoring your liver health, many of the supplements and nutrients discussed in this chapter can be vital. Antioxidants fight against disease-causing free radicals and can help reverse the effects of acetaminophen overdose. Herbs like milk thistle and turmeric have been used for thousands of years to protect liver cells from toxins. Probiotics are beneficial for their anti-inflammatory properties, while many vitamins and minerals contribute to your overall health.

While these supplements can all be purchased without a prescription, it is very important to discuss the use of any supplement with your physician first. You should also be sure to read the labels on your supplements. Some can interact with your medications or with each other, while others need to be taken in only a small amount to be effective.

11

Developing an Exercise Plan

dopting a healthy lifestyle is the first step to improving your liver health. A healthy lifestyle involves the maintenance of a nutritious diet and the utilization of supplements, which I reviewed in Chapters 9 and 10. Another important part of a healthy lifestyle is the development of an exercise plan. Whether your exercise of choice is walking, running, swimming, biking, yoga, or something else, just thirty minutes a day of any activity is sufficient to sustain your wellbeing.

If you have liver disease, you may feel exhausted much of the time. It may seem counterintuitive or impossible to exercise when you feel so fatigued. However, exercise has been demonstrated to improve energy levels and help you sleep better at night. When combined with a healthy diet, exercise helps you lose fat (which is especially important for conditions such as non-alcoholic fatty liver disease) and gain muscle (which can counteract the muscle wasting that sometimes occurs in advanced liver disease). Exercise gives your metabolism a boost, and can help to regulate your blood sugar levels. Your cardiovascular health profits from exercise as well; exercise allows blood to flow more easily through the vessels that connect the liver to the rest of your body.

In this chapter, I will review two types of exercise (aerobic and resistance) and explain how each can benefit your liver health. Keep in mind that the significant health benefits of exercise occur most prominently in the preventive phase or if only a mild liver illness is present. If you have advanced liver disease or cirrhosis, it may be difficult to fully participate in an exercise program. Consult with your doctor before beginning an exercise program to ensure that it poses no risk to your heart.

HOW EXERCISE BENEFITS THE LIVER

You may already know many of the health advantages that exercise can provide you, such as weight loss and muscle growth. However, as somebody with liver disease, you may be wondering how exercise can help your liver specifically. The following sections cover a few of exercise's many beneficial effects on the liver.

Balances Blood Sugar

Many people have liver disease alongside metabolic syndrome. Metabolic syndrome is a group of symptoms that predispose a person to developing heart disease or liver disease, especially NAFLD and non-alcoholic steatohepatitis (NASH). High blood sugar and high cholesterol levels are included in metabolic syndrome. Exercise can be helpful for managing these conditions.

For example, exercising can increase insulin sensitivity, which lowers high blood sugar by helping the cell utilize glucose more efficiently. Exercise can improve many of the complications that may occur with diabetes, such as by relieving fatigue, strengthening flexibility and bone health, and reducing stress or depression. If you have diabetes, consult with your doctor before beginning an exercise program, as you may need to adjust your food intake.

Reduces Cholesterol Levels

Exercise has the ability to balance cholesterol levels, as well. A study performed at Duke University placed patients with high cholesterol into three different exercise groups; each group varied in terms of length and intensity of the exercise. A fourth group did not exercise. The participants followed their exercise programs for six months, without changing their diets. The results found that higher amounts of exercise (regardless of intensity) caused the size of the protein particles that carry cholesterol to increase. (Larger particles have a lower chance of causing cardiovascular disease than do smaller particles.) Those who exercised saw an improvement in their levels of "good" HDL cholesterol, as well. The participants in the fourth, non-exercising group experienced weight gain and a worsening of their cholesterol levels.

Reduces Fatty Liver

As you learned in Chapter 3, NAFLD is the accumulation of fat cells in the liver. It is strongly correlated with obesity. Exercise (along with a balanced diet) can counteract obesity and its associated health risks. Many studies have demonstrated the preventative effects that exercise has on fatty liver development. One study followed patients with NASH as they complied with an exercise program. This program consisted of aerobic exercise (see page 172) for thirty minutes a day, five days a week. After three months, the patients who had stuck with the exercise program saw normalized liver enzymes and a slight drop in waist circumference and BMI (body mass index). Patients who had failed to follow through with the program saw no significant changes in their liver enzymes.

It is important to note that too rapid of a weight loss can worsen NAFLD; if you start an exercise routine and notice you are losing weight very quickly, consider easing the intensity or length of the program.

BASICS OF EXERCISE

Now that you know some of the benefits that exercise can provide your liver, where do you begin when creating an exercise plan? There are two main types of exercise: aerobic exercise (which builds up endurance) and resistance training (which builds up muscle strength). Aerobic training is "cardio" exercise and can include activities such as walking or swimming. Resistance training is strength training; think of weightlifting or push-ups. Resistance training is especially important to consider if you have advanced liver disease (see inset on page 172).

Before beginning any exercise program, it is important to first talk with your doctor. Some risk factors and symptoms of liver disease can affect your heart. For example, diabetes is a condition that is commonly linked to fatty liver. Diabetes is also a risk factor for heart disease. Alcohol consumption is also toxic to the heart (in addition to being a toxin to the liver and muscles). It has been associated with the development of heart muscle disease, or *cardiomyopathy*, and (in some instances) can contribute to abnormal rhythms of the heart (*arrhythmias*).

Exercise can alleviate these conditions, but it can be stressful to your heart, especially if you are already susceptible to heart disease. Speak with your doctor about your specific risk factors and medical history to determine if it is safe for you to start an exercise program.

Resistance Training and Advanced Liver Disease

In this chapter, you learn about aerobic exercise and resistance training. While aerobic exercise is very beneficial in the preventative stage or in cases of mild liver disease, resistance training is especially important to your liver health if you have an advanced disease. This is because an advanced condition can cause *muscle atrophy,* or weakening of the muscles, over time. The longer you have had an ill liver, the greater your risk of developing muscle atrophy. If you heavily drink alcohol, this puts you at a higher risk for both muscle atrophy and muscle *myopathy.* Muscle myopathy is an inflammatory response in the muscles, whereas atrophy is a loss of mass and strength. Myopathy can happen more acutely (suddenly) than atrophy. Stopping alcohol consumption is one important component of maintaining both liver and muscle strength. Adding resistance training builds your muscles up and makes them stronger, so your muscles will not be extremely weakened and your risk of developing atrophy will be decreased.

Aerobic Exercise

Aerobic exercise increases your body's endurance and strengthens the heart. There are many types of aerobic exercise that you may like to participate in. A few of them are listed below:

- **Biking.** Biking is a great exercise, especially if you have bad knees or arthritis, as there is less impact on the joints than there is in activities such as running. You can use a stationary bike (which may be easier because of its adjustable settings) or ride a bicycle outside (allowing you some fresh air and sunlight). If you use a stationary bike, I recommend using one that allows you to move the arms back and forth in addition to the legs; this works all muscle groups.

- **Swimming.** Swimming is an excellent fat-burning exercise that works muscles in the arms and legs. It is also a good choice if you have arthritis, because it has a very low impact on your joints. You will need to have access to a pool, or an outdoor body of water if you are an experienced swimmer. In any setting, make sure there is a lifeguard nearby in case of a medical emergency. If you are just embarking on a swimming program, take alternate days off so that your muscles can recover. An alternative to swimming is aqua therapy, which consists of movements such as walking or running in the water.

- **Walking.** Walking is one of the best and easiest exercises you can engage in, especially if you have never exercised before. It is also low-impact and will not wear and tear your muscles. Even walking for thirty minutes a day has health benefits. If you are walking indoors on a treadmill, start by walking on a flat incline at low speed. You can then slowly increase the incline and walking speed.

Resistance Training

Ideally, you will want to alternate a day of aerobic exercise with a day of resistance training. Resistance-based exercise typically consists of using circuit training machines or lifting free weights.

Here are some general tips for resistance training:

- Start with a weight with which you can complete five repetitions comfortably. Wait sixty seconds before starting the next set. You want to slowly increase to up to ten repetitions per set for each exercise.

- Circuit-based training machines are a little different from lifting free weights. There are a number of machines that work different muscle groups. During a circuit, you usually use seven to ten machines, doing one to two sets on each. A circuit typically lasts at least thirty minutes. I recommend waiting until you have built up some endurance first (using free weights) before starting a circuit-based regimen; ask your doctor if you are not sure.

- It is best to target different muscle groups on different days. For example, do arm workouts one day, core workouts the next time, and leg workouts the next time. This prevents any one area from becoming too fatigued during the week.

Preventing Injury

When you begin a program, you may be eager to start your workout right away. However, it is important to take some steps to prevent injury. If you join a gym, be sure that you speak with one of the personal trainers during your first visit, especially if you have never used the equipment before. This is particularly important if you will be doing weight and resistance training; using the proper techniques decreases the risk of injury. The gym staff can teach you the correct form for weightlifting and how to properly use different machines.

Some other tips that you should keep in mind are the following:

- Warming up first is important in preventing muscle injury. For example, if you will be doing aerobic exercise, you should walk for two to five minutes beforehand. Or, if you will be using a stationary bike, pedal against low resistance for five minutes first.

- After warming up your muscles, it is important to stretch them. Stretching improves your flexibility and range of motion. The muscles should be warmed up before you stretch to reduce the risk of injury.

- When you start your specific exercise, start slow and gradually increase your time and intensity over a number of weeks. This is especially important if you are doing aerobic exercise. You do not want to over-exert yourself and fatigue your body.

- If this is the first time that you have begun an exercise program, or if it has been a long time since you last exercised, it will take time for your body to adapt. Do not become discouraged if you cannot immediately complete an exercise—you will get there in time! Listen to your body when it begins to tire. Take at least one or two rest days a week to allow your body to recover.

OTHER FORMS OF EXERCISE

While there is evidence to support the roles that aerobic and resistance exercises have in liver health, they are not the only ways to get a workout. Gyms and machines are not everybody's cup of tea. The good news is that any active movement can benefit your health. There are many alternative forms of exercise, such as yoga, which can bring you to a state of relaxation while still strengthening your muscles and flexibility. Even a hobby that does not seem like exercise, such as gardening, can improve your cardiovascular health because you are constantly moving. Talk with your doctor about the activities you do on a daily basis to evaluate if any additional exercise is recommended for you.

SUPPLEMENTING YOUR EXERCISE PROGRAM

In the last chapter, you read about liver-friendly nutritional supplements. If you are beginning an exercise program, I believe that there are several other supplements that can benefit you. These supplements can help your muscles recover from your workouts; they help the muscles work more efficiently and can provide more energy to them. The combination of all three of the following supplements really assists in muscle recovery; however, just taking an individual one can be beneficial as well. Many people will begin with one and wait a few weeks to see how they are doing before adding a second one. These supplements include:

- **Coenzyme Q10 (CoQ10).** An antioxidant that is made by your body naturally; it functions as a vitamin, as well. It is thought to protect the muscles from exercise-induced injury. Some data suggests that CoQ10 may increase your ability to exercise for a longer time, which is significant—especially given the muscle fatigue that can occur in chronic and advanced liver disease (see inset on page 172). I recommend a dose of 100 milligrams, taken twice a day.

- **D-ribose.** Also known as simply "ribose," this is a sugar that is naturally produced by the body as an energy source. It can prevent the muscles from becoming too fatigued during exercise. A study found that those who supplemented with 10 grams of ribose a day before a workout experienced a significant increase in work performed and in strength while bench pressing, compared to a placebo group that performed the same workout. I recommend you start with a minimum dose of 2,500 milligrams a day.

- **L-carnitine.** This is an amino acid that is naturally produced by the body. Supplementing with L-carnitine can be an effective way to recover from exercise. For example, one study found that those who used 2,000 milligrams of L-carnitine before exercising had less than half of the muscle disruption of those who used a placebo. The subjects who used L-carnitine also had much lower ratings in muscle soreness. It can be used to increase athletic endurance, as well. I recommend a dose starting at 500 mg taken twice a day.

SUMMARY

Along with the diet adjustments and supplementary therapy that are described in Chapters 9 and 10, adopting an exercise program is an essential part of keeping you and your liver healthy. Exercise helps relieve the symptoms of metabolic disorder (including high blood sugar and high cholesterol levels) and can decrease the fatigue, stress, and depression you may be experiencing after being diagnosed with liver disease. Incorporating both aerobic exercise and weight-resistance types of exercise is important. However, any activity that gets you moving is beneficial to your health. Supplementation with key nutrients can help you recover from your workouts more quickly. Keep in mind that your goal is not necessarily to lose weight (although this can relieve some symptoms)—the goal is to decrease the number of fat cells within your liver.

The most important part of exercising is to find activities that you truly enjoy doing! If you like what you are doing, you are more likely to make it a part of your daily routine, which will lead to a happier and healthier lifestyle.

Conclusion

opefully, this book has been able to answer many of the questions you may have had. As a doctor, it is all too common to see patients overcome with emotion when they are told about an unexpected diagnosis. What I try to make clear is that whether someone is a patient or caretaker, the more they know, the better prepared they will be to make informed decisions—for them, knowledge is power. For you, it is as well.

In this book, you read about the many important responsibilities your liver has in your health. The liver processes the substances you consume and provides nutrients to the rest of your body, while eliminating toxic materials. It produces proteins, balances your blood sugar levels, clots the blood, and helps regulate your immune system, among other functions. Having a healthy liver is necessary for living.

If you or a loved one has been diagnosed with liver disease, it can come as a shock—especially because in many cases, few or no symptoms have been present. By now, you have learned that liver disease is not something that can be ignored. Often, the liver is not the only organ harmed by liver disease; the kidneys and the brain can become affected if the liver disease advances. In this book, we have discussed the most well-known and common liver diseases: viral hepatitis (types A, B, and C), cirrhosis, nonalcoholic fatty liver disease (NAFLD) and nonalcoholic steatohepatitis (NASH), and liver cancer. There are many potential causes for each of these conditions, including contamination by infected substances, inherited disorders, or external circumstances (such as heavy alcohol or drug consumption).

If you suspect that you have liver disease, there are a number of examinations your doctor can perform. With early intervention, it is possible to restore your liver health, whether that is through eliminating alcohol, cutting down on over-the-counter drugs (especially acetamino-phen), changing your diet, or adding nutritional supplements.

In cases of advanced and chronic liver disease, further steps will need to be taken. You may need to be evaluated for a liver transplant, or under-go a medication program. It may feel overwhelming to see multiple doc-tors. My goal when writing this book has been to simplify this process and explain the examinations, health care professionals, and treatments that are available to you. It is my hope that you come away from this book with an appreciation for the liver's importance and an understanding of how to best manage your condition.

Now that you have been armed with the basic information about liver disease, the next step is to start actively combating it. Talk with your doc-tor about the best medication options for you. Learn more about your pre-scriptions. Consider a slow liver detoxification. Review your diet and exercise habits and see if there are any positive changes you can make. Look into herbal and supplementary treatments, as long as they do not conflict with your medication. If you are on the waiting list for a liver transplant, spend some time learning about the process and preparing for your hospital stay (this includes deciding who will be your caretaker dur-ing the recovery period). Ask your doctor any and all questions you can think of. Remember that while doctors can assist and advise you, ulti-mately, you are the one who is responsible for your own health. Being proactive in your care is the first step toward real change.

Liver disease can be a debilitating and frightening condition—but it doesn't *have* to be. With the help of this book and your family, friends, and health care providers, you can start down the road toward a happy and healthy liver.

Glossary

Albumin. Albumin is the most dominant protein circulating in the blood; it is produced in the liver. Low levels can suggest poor nutrition or medical conditions, including liver and kidney disease; it is used as a marker of nutritional status by many health professionals.

Alcoholic hepatitis. This refers to the acute inflammation of the liver due to excessive alcohol consumption.

Ammonia. Ammonia is a toxic byproduct that is produced when the liver is not able to effectively metabolize protein. Ammonia buildup can cause hepatic encephalopathy in someone with advanced liver disease.

Antioxidants. Defensive molecules in the body, such as vitamin C and glutathione, that neutralize the damage done by free radicals.

Ascites. Ascites is the accumulation of fluid in the abdominal cavity. This is due to portal hypertension and it is a common sign that liver disease may be present. Cirrhosis is a leading cause of ascites. (See also *portal hypertension.*)

Bile. This is a brownish liquid produced by the liver that is transported to the gallbladder and intestines. It has several functions, such as helping the body digest food.

Child-Pugh score. This is a classification score that is used to determine the extent and severity of liver disease.

Cirrhosis. Cirrhosis is an advanced, chronic liver disease that is often irreversible. It is characterized by scarring in the liver cells. Its presence can be detected on imaging studies (such as an ultrasound); a cirrhotic liver will often appear small and shrunken. Chronic alcohol use, fatty liver, and hepatitis B and C are common causes of cirrhosis.

Cirrhotic cardiomyopathy. An abnormal heart condition that is felt to be due to cirrhosis.

Coagulation factors. Also known as "clotting factors," these are produced by the liver to clot the blood. A diseased liver may have a decreased ability to produce these, leading to a higher risk of excessive bleeding.

Detoxification. The process of eliminating toxic substances from the liver to cleanse the body.

Diuretics. This is a class of medications that manage swelling due to excess fluid buildup (ascites or edema).

Edema. Excess fluid and swelling in the legs or ankles. Edema can be a sign of heart disease, kidney disease, and/or liver disease. In liver disease, edema often co-occurs with ascites.

Epstein-Barr virus (EBV). This is the virus that causes mononucleosis, among other illnesses. This virus can also (less commonly) cause acute hepatitis.

Fatty liver. Fatty liver is the most common cause of liver disease. It is an accumulation of fat cells in the liver. A liver is considered to be fatty if more than 5 to 10 percent of its weight is fat. This term can also be used in a general way to refer to non-alcoholic fatty liver disease (NAFLD), in which there is fat deposition but no acute inflammation, or non-alcoholic steatohepatitis (NASH), in which there is acute inflammation.

Ferritin. This is a protein produced by the liver. It is important for storing, regulating, and releasing iron into the body.

Free radicals. These are unstable molecules in the body that are highly reactive and can cause cell damage.

Fulminant hepatitis. An uncommon condition in which the liver's health deteriorates rapidly.

Gastroenterologist. A doctor who specializes in treatment of the gastrointestinal (GI), or digestive, system. Gastroenterologists also treat liver disease.

Hemochromatosis. A hereditary condition in which too much iron is stored in the body.

Hepatic encephalopathy. A condition in which the liver cannot properly remove toxins from the bloodstream, due to the buildup of ammonia. These toxins build up in the brain, causing cognitive decline.

Hepatitis. This refers to inflammation of the liver (either acute or chronic) and is characterized by an elevation in liver enzymes. There are many causes of hepatitis, including certain viruses, medications, alcohol, and fatty liver disease.

Hepatocellular carcinoma. The most common type of liver cancer.

Hepatocytes. These are cells that make up about 75 percent of the cells in the liver. They carry out many of the liver's most important functions.

Hepatologist. A doctor who has received specialized training in matters of the liver.

Hepatomegaly. An enlarged liver.

Hepatorenal syndrome. A condition in which kidney function is compromised due to liver disease.

Jaundice. This refers to the yellowing of the skin and eyes, caused by a buildup of bile. It is a common initial sign of liver disease.

Kupffer cells. These are cells in the liver that clean blood of bacteria, fungi, parasites, and other harmful materials.

Liver function tests. These are blood tests that check the levels of these enzymes: albumin, alkaline phosphatase, alanine aminotransferase (ALT), aspartate aminotransferase (AST), and total bilirubin. Measurements of these enzymes can indicate if the liver is functioning adequately.

Liver transplant. A surgery in which a healthy liver is given to a patient with liver disease. This can be achieved through cadaveric donation (in which the liver donor has recently passed away) or living donation (in which a portion of a living person's liver is transplanted).

MELD (Model for End-Stage Liver Disease) score. This is a classification score that is used to determine if a patient is eligible to obtain a liver transplant.

Non-alcoholic fatty liver disease (NAFLD). Deposition of excess fat in the liver without the presence of hepatitis.

Non-alcoholic steatohepatitis (NASH). This is a severe subset of NAFLD. It is characterized by an inflammation in the liver due to fat deposition.

Oxidative stress. This is an imbalance of free radicals and antioxidants in the body.

Palpation. This refers to the method a doctor may use to initially check for signs of an enlarged liver. It involves pressing around your right-hand side rib cage.

Paracentesis. This is a procedure performed by a physician or health care professional in which excess fluid caused by ascites is removed.

Portal hypertension. This refers to a buildup of pressure in the liver. Think of this as being the equivalent of "high blood pressure in the liver." Complications of elevated portal hypertension include internal bleeding, such as esophageal varices.

Viral hepatitis. This condition causes inflammation in the liver. Common causes of viral hepatitis include the hepatitis A, B, or C viruses. Hepatitis viruses can be contagious.

Wilson's disease. A hereditary condition in which an excess of copper is stored in the body.

Resources

There is a vast network of support for those who have liver disease. There are a significant number of websites and organizations that can provide you with excellent information concerning liver health and liver disease. In addition, in this section you will find resources for locating physicians, specialists, and alternative and integrative health care providers.

LIVER-BASED INFORMATION WEBSITES

American Association for the Study of Liver Diseases (AASLD)
1001 North Fairfax Street, Suite 400
Alexandria, VA 22314
Phone: (703) 299-9766
Website: www.aasld.org
This is a national organization that is dedicated to health professionals and scientists. It provides up-to-date information and research on liver health and liver disease. The AASLD's goal is to provide health care professionals with the knowledge needed to prevent and cure liver disease.

American Liver Foundation
39 Broadway, Suite 2700
New York, NY 10006
Phone: (212) 668-1000
Helpline: (800) 465-4837
Website: www.liverfoundation.org
This is a national organization aimed for patients who have liver disease and their families. The objective of this site is noted on its mission statement: To "facilitate, advocate, and promote education, support, and research for the prevention, treatment, and cure of liver disease." Educational resources and services are provided, including webinars concerning various aspects of liver disease. In addition, the site provides a national helpline to answer questions concerning liver health.

Hepatitis B Foundation
3805 Old Easton Road
Doylestown, PA 18902
Phone: (215) 489-4900
Website: www.hepb.org
This is a national organization whose goal is education and research regarding the treatment of hepatitis B. The organization also provides support for those who have this condition.

Hepatitis C Association
1351 Cooper Road
Scotch Plains, NJ 07076
Phone: (877) 435-7443
Website: www.hepcassoc.org
This is a national organization that provides education and information specifically about hepatitis C. The website covers topics such as risk factors, prevention, and treatment of this condition. This site is meant for both medical professionals and the public.

Hepatitis Foundation International
8121 Georgia Avenue, Suite 350
Silver Spring, MD 20910
Phone: (800) 891-0707
Website: www.hepatitisfoundation
.org
This is a national non-profit organization whose goal is to educate the public in topics of "liver wellness and healthy lifestyles" to prevent conditions, such as diabetes and obesity, that can develop into liver disease. This website provides helpful resources, such as DVDs and a phone hotline.

FINDING INTEGRATIVE HEALTH PROVIDERS

American Academy of Anti-Aging Medicine
Phone: (888) 997-0112
Website: www.a4m.com;
www.worldhealth.net
This organization, nicknamed A4M, is a medical society comprising of over 26,000 health care professionals who have undergone a specialized fellowship in anti-aging medicine. A4M's goal is to provide information on age-related disease. To find a health care professional certified in anti-aging medicine near you, click on "Directory." You will then need to fill in more information, such as your zip code.

American Board of Integrative Holistic Medicine
Website: www.abihm.org
This is an organization whose practitioners embrace a holistic approach

to the treatment of disease, with an emphasis on health prevention and wellness. The website provides a search engine with which you can look for a holistic medicine-based physician in your area.

National Center For Homeopathy
7918 Jones Branch Drive, Suite 300
McLean, VA 22102
Phone: (703) 506-7667
Website: www.homeopathic.org
This is a national organization that provides educational resources and information for both homeopathic practitioners and the public. Its goal is to inform the public, the health care system, and the media of homeopathic care and ensure its accessibility. You can also use the website to find a homeopathic practitioner in or near your area.

FINDING TRADITIONAL PHYSICIANS AND LIVER SPECIALISTS

Doctors.At
Website: www.doctors.at
This site allows you to search for physicians by specialty and state. One can search for complementary and alternative medicine providers, as well.

Hepatitis B Foundation Liver Specialist Directory
Website: www.hepb.org/resources/
liver-specialist-state-list.htm

This is a service provided by the Hepatitis B Foundation (see above) and is an excellent resource for patients who wish to search for a liver specialist. Just click on the state of interest, and liver specialists from that state will appear. It provides information such as affiliations, approximate patient loads, and if the practitioner speaks languages other than English.

ALCOHOLISM REHABILITATION

Alcoholics Anonymous
Phone: (212) 870-3400
Website: www.aa.org
Alcoholics Anonymous is the largest twelve-step program in the nation. It is comprised of volunteers who are dedicated to helping alcoholics recover from their addiction. The focus is placed on casual but therapeutic discussions.

Recovery.org
Phone: (888) 319-2606
Website: www.recovery.org
This website's mission is to link people who have addictions (including to alcohol and drugs) to over 8,000 programs and resources to aid them in their recovery. The website also provides a hotline that patients can call to speak with a counselor.

NATURAL SUPPLEMENTS

BioInnovations
Phone: (888) 442-6161
Website: www.bioinnovations.net
This is a company that offers many natural products, including probiotics and other supplements, that benefit the liver and total body health. BioInnovations also carries books and other educational resources.

LifeTime Vitamins
Phone: (800) 333-6168
Website: www.lifetimevitamins.com
Lifetime Vitamins carries natural vitamins; in addition, they also carry plant-based protein powders to provide nutritional support, as discussed in Chapter 8. The website provides information on the various supplements and powders available.

NUTRITIONAL PLANNING AND ORGANIC FOOD

Celiac Disease Foundation
Website: www.celiac.org

As mentioned in Chapter 9, celiac disease and cirrhosis can go hand-in-hand. Even if you do not have celiac disease, following a gluten-free diet can provide some benefits. This website provides information about celiac disease and support for those who have it.

The DASH Diet Eating Plan
Website: www.dashdiet.org

In Chapter 9, I explained the benefits of following the DASH diet. The website for this diet provides many helpful resources, such as sample menus for vegetarians and non-vegetarians, grocery shopping tips, and information about other healthy diets (such as the Mediterranean diet).

Food For Life Baking Company
Phone: (800) 797-5090
Website: www.foodforlife.com

The Food for Life Baking Company carries all-natural goods, including breads, cereal, pasta, and more. Their food products have been developed to satisfy certain dietary requirements, including gluten- and wheat-free as well as yeast-free foods.

Glycemic Index
Website: www.glycemicindex.com

This informative website, established by the University of Sydney in Australia, provides basic information concerning the glycemic index. The glycemic index measures how a food affects your blood sugar level. The website provides statistics on the glycemic index of many foods.

MyPlate
Website: www.livestrong.com/ myplate

This program allows members who register to track their daily calorie intake and exercise routines. It encourages and guides users to help achieve their ideal weight by providing a very simple way to track daily food consumption. Healthy dietary habits are emphasized.

Organic Valley Farms
Phone: (888) 444-6455
Website: www.organicvalley.coop

This is a national organization that utilizes a cooperative-style business model and depends on the efforts of member farmers all across the country. By clicking on "Who's Your Farmer?" on the website, you can locate Organic Valley farmers near you and order their products.

SELF Nutrition Data
Website: nutritiondata.self.com

Designed by a nutritionist for SELF Magazine, this comprehensive website serves as a database that provides nutritional information and analyses on any given food. It is also is a great educational resource; for example, it includes a page on reading food labels. You are able to track healthy recipes and develop your own personalized diet plan using the tools on the website.

TRANSPLANT CENTERS AND RESOURCES

Scientific Registry of Transplant Recipients (SRTR)

Website: www.srtr.org

This organization's website is a database of transplant-related information for both physicians and patients. Among its many roles, the website provides an up-to-date list of all liver transplant centers in the United States. Important statistics that you can find include the number of procedures a transplant center has performed, how many transplants were from a living donor or a deceased donor, and patient survival data.

United Network for Organ Sharing (UNOS)

Website: www.unos.org

UNOS manages the Organ Procurement and Transplantation Network (OPTN)— the nationwide organ transplant system. In addition, UNOS manages the waiting list for organ transplants and ensures that policies and procedures concerning the transplant process are followed. This organization's website is comprehensive and provides information detailing all aspects of the transplant process. There are dedicated topic sections for both the health professional and the patient.

References

CHAPTER 1

Andrews, R. "All About Cholesterol: Understanding nutrition's most controversial molecule." *PrecisionNutrition.* www.precisionnutrition.com/all-about-cholesterol

Belsley, S. "The Role of the Liver in Digestion." *Laparoscopic.md.* Accessed Nov. 16, 2015. www.laparoscopic.md/digestion/liver

Informed Health Online. "How does the liver work?" *PubMed Health.* Last modified Nov. 22, 2012. www.ncbi.nlm.nih.gov/pubmedhealth/PMH0072577/

Lechner, K, et al. "Coagulation abnormalities in liver disease." *Seminars in Thrombosis and Hemostasis* 1977; 4(1):40–56.

Losser, MR, and D Payen. "Mechanisms of Liver Damage." *Seminars in Liver Disease* 1996; 16(4):357–367.

Robinson, J. "Understanding Gallstones—The Basics." *WebMD.* Last modified March 7, 2015. www.webmd.com/digestive-disorders/gallstones-directory

Sawchenko, PE, and MI Friedman. "Sensory functions of the liver—a review." *American Journal of Physiology* 1979; 236(1):R5–R20.

Taylor, T. "Anatomy of the Liver." *InnerBody.com.* Accessed Nov. 16, 2015. www.innerbody.com/image_digeov/card10-new2.html

Winsor, S. "The Liver: Anatomy and Functions." *University of Rochester Medical Center.* Accessed Nov. 16, 2015. https://www.urmc.rochester.edu/encyclopedia/content.aspx?ContentTypeID=85&ContentID=P00676

CHAPTER 2

Afdhal, NH, et al. "Accuracy of fibroscan, compared with histology, in analysis of liver fibrosis in patients with hepatitis B or C: a United States multicenter study." *Clinical Gastroenterology and Hepatology* 2015; 13(4):772–779.

Afzali, A, et al. "Association between serum uric acid level and chronic liver disease in the United States." *Hepatology* 2010; 52(2):578–589.

"Blood tests for liver function." *Liver Doctor.* Accessed Dec.10, 2015. www.liverdoctor.com/liver/liver-function-tests/

Bolognesi, M, et al. "Role of spleen enlargement in cirrhosis with portal hypertension." *Digestive and Liver Disease* 2002; 34(2):144–150.

Chow, J and C Chow. *The Encyclopedia of Hepatitis and Other Liver Diseases.* New York: Facts on File, Inc., 2006.

Desmet, VJ, et al. "Classification of chronic hepatitis: diagnosis, grading and staging." *Hepatology* 1994; 19(6):1513–1520.

Drebber, U, et al. "The role of Epstein-Barr virus in acute and chronic hepatitis." *Journal of Hepatology* 2006; 44(5):879–885.

Foreman, MG, DM Mannino, and M Moss. "Cirrhosis as a risk factor for sepsis and death: analysis of the National Hospital Discharge Survey." *Chest* 2003; 124(3):1016–1020.

HealthLiving Staff. "8 Common Signs of Liver Damage." *HealthLiving.today.* Last modified May 2015. http://healthliving.today/physical-health/8-common-signs-of-liver-damage/

"Hepatitis." *Aria Health.* Accessed Dec. 10, 2015. https://www.ariahealth.org/programs-and-services/gastrointestinal-disease/hepatitis

Herrine, S. "Portal Hypertension." *Merck Manual.* Last modified July 2014. www.merck-manuals.com/professional/hepatic-and-biliary-disorders/approach-to-the-patient-with-liver-disease/portal-hypertension

Hoofnagle, JH. "Hepatitis C: the clinical spectrum of disease." *Hepatology* 1997; 26(3 Suppl 1):15S–20S.

Johnston, D. "Special Considerations in Interpreting Liver Function Tests." *American Family Physician* 1999; 59(8): 2223–2230.

Runyon, BA, et al. "The serum-ascites albumin gradient is superior to the exudates-transudate concept in the differential diagnosis of ascites." *Annals of Internal Medicine* 1992; 117(3):215–220.

"What is hepatitis?" *World Health Organization.* Last modified July 2015. www.who.int/features/qa/76/en/

CHAPTER 3

Adams, LA, and P Angulo. "Treatment of non-alcoholic fatty liver disease." *Postgraduate Medical Journal* 2006; 82: 315–322.

Aspinall, EJ, et al. "Hepatitis B prevention, diagnosis, treatment and care: a review." *Occupational Medicine* 2011; 61(8):531–540.

Chayanupatkul, M, and S Liangpunsakul. "Alcoholic hepatitis: a comprehensive review of pathogenesis and treatment." *World Journal of Gastroenterology* 2014; 20(20): 6279–6286.

"Cirrhosis." *National Institute of Diabetes and Digestive and Kidney Diseases.* Last modified April 2014. www.niddk.nih.gov/health-information/health-topics/liver-disease/cirrhosis/Pages/facts.aspx

"Donating Blood." *Hepatitis B Foundation.* Last modified Feb. 2014. www.hepb.org/hepb/blood_donations.htm

Ewing, JA. "Detecting alcoholism. The CAGE questionnaire." *JAMA* 1984; 252(14):1905–1907.

Gilroy, R. "Wilson disease." *MedScape.* Last modified Jan. 11, 2016. http://emedicine.medscape.com/article/183456-overview

Gunsar, F. "Treatment of delta hepatitis." *Expert Review of Anti-infective Therapy* 2013; 11(5): 489–498.

Haché, C, and JP Villeneuve. "Lamivudine treatment in patients with chronic hepatitis B and cirrhosis." *Expert Opinion on Pharmacotherapy* 2006; 7(13): 1835–1843.

Hannuksela, J, et al. "Hereditary hemochromatosis gene (HFE) mutations C282Y, H63D and S65C in patients with idiopathic dilated cardiomyopathy." *European Journal of Heart Failure* 2005; 7(1): 103–108.

"Hepatitis A." *The New York Times.* Last modified Oct. 13, 2013. www.nytimes.com/health/guides/disease/hepatitis-a/overview.html

"Hepatitis C testing." *HepMag.* Last modified Jan. 11, 2016. www.hepmag.com/articles/2951_18753.shtml

"Hepatitis C testing for anyone born during 1945–1965: New CDC recommendations." *Centers for Disease Control and Prevention.* Last modified Oct. 1, 2012. www.cdc.gov/features/HepatitisCTesting/

Jepsen, P, and H Gronbaek. "Prognosis and staging of non-alcoholic fatty liver disease." *BMJ* 2011; 343: d7302.

Karlas, T, et al. "Estimating steatosis and fibrosis: Comparison of acoustic structure quantification with established techniques." *World Journal of Gastroenterology* 2015; 21(16): 4894–4902.

Kinoshita, A, et al. "Staging systems for hepatocellular carcinoma: Current status and future perspectives." *World Journal of Hepatology* 2015; 7(3): 406–424.

Lima, LR, et al. "Evidence of hepatitis A virus person-to-person transmission in household outbreaks." *PLoS One* 2014; 9(7).

Lin, CL, and JH Kao. "Hepatitis B virus genotypes and variants." *Cold Spring Harbor Perspectives in Medicine* 2015; 5(5): a021436.

"Liver Cancer." *American Cancer Society.* www.cancer.org/cancer/livercancer/index

"Liver Cancer." *American Liver Foundation.* Last modified Nov. 6, 2015. www.liverfoundation.org/abouttheliver/info/livercancer

Mayo Clinic staff. "Alcoholic hepatitis." *Mayo Clinic.* Last modified Nov. 25, 2015. www.mayoclinic.org/diseases-conditions/alcoholic-hepatitis/home/ovc-20163921

Mayo Clinic staff. "Cirrhosis." *Mayo Clinic.* Last modified Aug. 16, 2014. www.mayoclinic.org/diseases-conditions/cirrhosis/basics/definition/con-20031617

Mayo Clinic staff. "Hemochromatosis." *Mayo Clinic.* Last modified Dec. 22, 2015. www.mayoclinic.org/diseases-conditions/hemochromatosis/basics/definition/con-20023606

Mayo Clinic staff. "Nonalcoholic fatty liver disease." *Mayo Clinic.* Last modified April 10, 2014. www.mayoclinic.org/diseases-conditions/nonalcoholic-fatty-liver-disease/basics/symptoms/con-20027761

Mederacke, I, et al. "Renal function during treatment with adefovir plus peginterferon alfa-2a vs either drug alone in hepatitis B/D co-infection." *Journal of Viral Hepatitis* 2012; 19(6): 387–395.

"NAFLD." *American Liver Foundation.* Last modified Jan. 14, 2015. www.liverfoundation.org/abouttheliver/info/nafld/

Nam, TH, et al. "Non-invasive assessment of liver fibrosis using acoustic structure quantification: comparison with transient elastography in chronic viral hepatitis." *Abdominal Radiology* 2016; 41(2): 239–247.

Polo, D, MF Varela, and JL Romalde. "Detection and quantification of hepatitis A virus and norovirus in Spanish authorized shellfish harvesting areas." *International Journal of Food Microbiology* 2015; 193:43–50.

Ranucci, G, et al. "Zinc monotherapy is effective in Wilson's disease patients with mild liver disease diagnosed in childhood: a retrospective study." *Orphanet Journal of Rare Disease* 2014; 9: 41.

Roche, B, and D Samuel. "Liver transplantation in delta virus infection." *Seminars in Liver Disease* 2012; 32(3): 245–255.

Sertoglu, E, et al. "The relationship of serum uric acid with non-alcoholic fatty liver disease." *Clinical Biochemistry* 2014; 47(6): 383–388.

Shaukat, A, et al. "Epstein-Barr virus induced hepatitis: An important cause of cholestasis." *Hepatology Research* 2005; 33(1): 24–26.

Shepherd, J, et al. "Adefovir dipivoxil and pegylated interferon alfa-2a for the treatment of hepatitis B: a systematic review and economic evaluation." *Health Technology Assessment* 2006; 10(28):iii–iv, xi–xiv, 1–183.

Siafakas, CG, et al. "Early onset of nephrotic syndrome after treatment with D-penicillamine in a patient with Wilson's disease." *American Journal of Gastroenterology* 1998; 93(12): 2544–2546.

Singal AK, and SC Jampana. "Current management of alcoholic liver disease." *Current Drug Abuse Reviews* 2014; 7(1):18–28.

Takeda, A, et al. "A systematic review and economic evaluation of adefovir dipivoxil and pegylated interferon-alpha-2a for the treatment of chronic hepatitis B." *Journal of Viral Hepatitis* 2007; 14(2): 75–88.

"Understanding Hepatitis B Blood Tests." *Hepatitis B Foundation.* Accessed Dec. 12, 2015. www.hepb.org/pdf/understanding_blood_tests.pdf

"Viral Hepatitis—Hepatitis C Information." *Centers for Disease Control and Prevention.* Last modified March 11, 2016. www.cdc.gov/hepatitis/hcv/hcvfaq.htm

Williams, CD, et al. "Prevalence of nonalcoholic fatty liver disease and nonalcoholic steatohepatitis among a largely middle-aged population utilizing ultrasound and liver biopsy: a prospective study." *Gastroenterology* 2011; 140(1):124–131.

Wong, LL, et al. "Liver transplant for hepatocellular cancer: A treatment for the select few." *Clinical Transplantation* 2004; 18(2): 205–210.

Zhou, X, et al. "Epidemiology and management of chronic hepatitis E infection in solid organ transplantation: a comprehensive literature review." *Reviews in Medical Virology* 2013; 23(5): 295–304.

CHAPTER 4

Adekanle, O, et al. "Cognitive functions in patients with liver cirrhosis: assessment using community screening interview for dementia." *Annals of African Medicine* 2012; 11(4):222–229.

"Adrenal Exhaustion." *Liver Doctor.* June 24, 2015. https://www.liverdoctor.com/adrenal-exhaustion/

Devuni, D. "Hepatorenal syndrome." *MedScape.* Last modified Jan. 13, 2016. http://emedicine.medscape.com/article/178208-overview

Fede, G, et al. "Adrenocortical dysfunction in liver disease: a systematic review." *Hepatology* 2012; 55(4):1282–1291.

Gines, A, et al. "Incidence, predictive factors, and prognosis of the hepatorenal syndrome in cirrhosis with ascites." *Gastroenterology* 1993; 105(1): 229–236.

Isobe, H, et al. "Delayed gastric emptying in patients with liver cirrhosis." *Digestive Diseases and Sciences* 1994; 39(5):983–987.

Lehrer, J. "Hepatorenal syndrome." *MedlinePlus.* Last updated May 15, 2014. www.nlm.nih.gov/medlineplus/ency/article/000489.htm

Marik, PE. "Adrenal-exhaustion syndrome in patients with liver disease." *Intensive Care Medicine* 2006; 32(2):275–280.

Marik, PE, et al. "The hepatoadrenal syndrome: a common yet unrecognized clinical condition." *Critical Care Medicine* 2005; 33(6):1254–1259.

Moller, S, and JH Henriksen. "Cirrhotic cardiomyopathy." *Journal of Hepatology* 2010; 53(1):179–190.

Moller, S, CW Dumcke, and A Krag. "The heart and the liver." *Expert Review of Gastroenterology and Hepatology* 2009; 3(1):51–64.

Sunmonu, TA, et al. "Cognitive function in patients with liver cirrhosis without overt hepatic encephalopathy: assessment using an automated neuropsychological test battery." *Arab Journal of Gastroenterology* 2012; 13(1):4–8.

Targher, G, et al. "Differences and similarities in early atherosclerosis between patients with non-alcoholic steatohepatitis and chronic hepatitis B and C." *Journal of Hepatology* 2007; 46(6): 1126–1132.

Verne, GN, et al. "Autonomic dysfunction and gastroparesis in cirrhosis." *Journal of Clinical Gastroenterology* 2004; 38(1):72–76.

CHAPTER 5

"Alcohol-Medication Interactions." *AlcoholScreening.org.* Accessed Jan. 5, 2016. www.alco-holscreening.org/Learn-More.aspx?topicID=8&articleID=37

Andrade, RJ, and PM Tulkens. "Hepatic safety of antibiotics used in primary care." *Journal of Antimicrobial Chemotherapy* 2011; 66(7): 1431–1446.

Andrade, SE, et al. "Liver function testing in patients on HMG-CoA reductase inhibitors." *Pharmacoepidemiology and Drug Safety* 2003; 12(4):307–313.

"Anticonvulsants." *LiverTox by National Institutes of Health.* Last modified March 24, 2016. http://livertox.nih.gov/AnticonvulsantDrugs.htm

Bhatt, D. "Why do I get a headache when I take my nitroglycerin?" *ABC News.* Nov. 24, 2008. http://abcnews.go.com/Health/HeartDiseaseLivingWith/story?id=4217596

"Comfrey." *LiverTox by National Institutes of Health.* Last modified March 24, 2016. http://livertox.nlm.nih.gov/Comfrey.htm

Fong, TL. "Dietary supplements can cause liver damage." *MedicineNet.* www.medi-cinenet.com/script/main/art.asp?articlekey=20320

Fontana, RJ. "Acute liver failure due to drugs." *Seminars in Liver Disease* 2008; 28(2): 175–187.

Fontana, RJ. "Acute liver failure including acetaminophen overdose." *Medical Clinics of North America* 2008; 92(4): 761–794.

Grant, LM, and DC Rockey. "Drug-induced liver injury." *Current Opinion in Gastroenterology* 2012; 28(3): 198–202.

Herrera, JL. "Medications and the liver." *American College of Gastroenterology.* Last modified Dec. 2012. http://patients.gi.org/topics/medications-and-the-liver/

Hinson, J, DW Roberts, and LP James. "Mechanisms of acetaminophen-induced liver necrosis." *Handbook of Experimental Pharmacology* 2010; 196: 369–405.

Knauf, H, and E Mutschler. "Liver cirrhosis with ascites: pathogenesis of resistance to di-uretics and long-term efficacy and safety of torasemide." *Cardiology* 1994; 84(Suppl 2):87–98.

Lancaster, EM, JR Hiatt, and A Zarrinpar. "Acetaminophen hepatotoxicity: an updated re-view." *Archives of Toxicology* 2015; 89(2):193–199.

Lee, D. "Drug-induced liver disease." *MedicineNet.* Last modified May 7, 2015. www.med-icinenet.com/drug_induced_liver_disease/page9.htm

"Liver Wellness: Increasing Public Awareness of Liver Health." *American Liver Foundation.* Accessed Jan. 5, 2016. www.liverfoundation.org/downloads/alf_download_614.pdf

Llamas, M. "FDA sets acetaminophen dose limit, warns of liver damage." *Drug Watch.* Jan. 28, 2014. www.drugwatch.com/2014/01/28/fda-limits-acetaminophen-liver-damage/

"Midodrine." *MedBroadcast.* Accessed Jan. 6, 2016. www.medbroadcast.com/drug/get-drug/Midodrine

"Nonsteroidal anti-inflammatory drugs." *LiverTox by National Institutes of Health.* Last modified March 24, 2016. http://livertox.nih.gov/NonsteroidalAntiinflammatoryDrugs.htm

Ogbru, O, and J Marks. "Isoniazid (Nydrazid, Laniazid, INH are all discontinued brands." *MedicineNet.* Last modified Feb. 11, 2015. www.medicinenet.com/isoniazid_inh/page2.htm

Perri, GA. "Ascites in patients with cirrhosis." *Canadian Family Physician* 2013; 59(12):1297–1299.

Phongsamran, PV, et al. "Pharmacotherapy for hepatic encephalopathy." *Drugs* 2010; 70(9):1131–1148.

Sarpong, E, and SH Zuvekas. "Statistical brief #458: Trends instating therapy among adults (age > 18), United States, 2000 to 2011." *Agency for Healthcare Research and Quality.* Nov. 2014. http://meps.ahrq.gov/mepsweb/data_files/publications/st458/stat458.shtml

Sharma, BC, et al. "A randomized, double-blind, controlled trial comparing rifaximin plus lactulose with lactulose alone in treatment of overt hepatic encephalopathy." *American Journal of Gastroenterology* 2013; 108(9): 1458–1463.

Wong, F, L Pantea, and K Sniderman. "Midodrine, octreotide, albumin, and TIPS in selected patients with cirrhosis and type 1 hepatorenal syndrome." *Hepatology* 2004; 40(1):55–64.

CHAPTER 6

American Academy of Physician Assistants. "Physician assistants in gastroenterology and hepatology." *Specialty Practice* 2010. https://www.aapa.org/WorkArea/DownloadAsset.aspx?id=623

Desai, AP, et al. "Co-management between hospitalist and hepatologist improves the quality of care of inpatients with chronic liver disease." *Journal of Clinical Gastroenterology* 2014; 48(4):e30–e36.

Michelfelder, AJ, KC Lee, and EM Bading. "Integrative medicine and gastrointestinal disease." *Primary Care* 2010; 37(2):255–267.

"What is a Gastroenterologist?" *American College of Gastroenterology.* Accessed Jan. 13, 2016. http://s3.gi.org/patients/ccrk/WhatIsAGastro.pdf

CHAPTER 7

American Liver Foundation. www.liverfoundation.org.

Brown, RS Jr. "Live donors in liver transplantation." *Gastroenterology* 2008; 134(6): 1802–1813.

Gehri, K. "Tips for transplant surgery/hospitalization." *Chopped Liver* (blog). Accessed Feb. 3, 2016. https://kkchoppedliver.wordpress.com/transplant-posts/tips-for-transplant-surgery/

Levy, GA, N Selzner, and DR Grant. "Fostering liver living donor liver transplantation." *Current Opinion in Organ Transplantation* 2016; 21(2): 224–230.

"Liver transplant guide." *University of Iowa Hospitals and Clinics.* Accessed Feb. 2, 2016. https://www.uihealthcare.org/otherservices.aspx?id=22620

"Liver transplant patient guide." *Keck School of Medicine of USC.* Accessed Feb. 2, 2016. www.surgery.usc.edu/hepatobiliary/pg-livertransplant-postoperativecomplications.html

"Liver transplant surgery." *Emory Healthcare.* Accessed Feb. 2, 2016. www.emoryhealthcare.org/transplant-liver/learn-about/surgery.html

"Liver transplantation." *National Institute of Diabetes and Digestive and Kidney Diseases.* April 2012. www.niddk.nih.gov/health-information/health-topics/liver-disease/liver-transplant/Pages/facts.aspx

"Living donor transplant surgery." *Baylor Health.* Accessed Feb. 2, 2016. www.baylortransplant.com/liver/livingdonor.html

Martin, P, et al. "Evaluation for liver transplantation in adults: 2013 practice guideline by the AASLD and the American Society of Transplantation." *American Association for the Study of Liver Diseases* 2013. https://www.aasld.org/sites/default/files/guideline_documents/evaluationadultltenhanced.pdf

"MELD and the waiting list for liver transplant." *California Pacific Medical Center.* Accessed Feb. 2, 2016. www.cpmc.org/advanced/liver/patients/topics/MELD.html

Newman, MB, and C Walter. "A case management journey through liver transplantation." Accessed Feb. 4, 2016. *Dorland Health.* www.dorlandhealth.com/dorland-health-articles/a-case-management-journey-through-liver-transplantation

Roayaie, K, and S Feng. "Liver transplantation." *University of California San Francisco.* Aug. 2008. http://transplant.surgery.ucsf.edu/conditions—procedures/liver-transplantation.aspx

Scientific Registry of Transplant Recipients. www.srtr.org.

United Network for Organ Sharing. www.unos.org.

CHAPTER 8

DiNicolantonio, JJ, JH O'Keefe, and SC Lucan. "An unsavory truth: sugar, more than salt, predisposes to hypertension and chronic disease." *American Journal of Cardiology* 2014; 114(7):1126–1128.

Environmental Protection Agency. "2014 TRI National Analysis: Executive Summary." *EPA.gov.* Jan. 2016. www.epa.gov/sites/production/files/2016-01/documents/2014-tri-na-exec-summary.pdf

Klein, AV, and H Kiat. "Detox diets for toxin elimination and weight management: a critical review of the evidence." *Journal of Human Nutrition and Dietetics* 2015; 28(6):675–686.

MacIntosh, A, and K Ball. "The effects of a short program of detoxification in disease-free individuals." *Alternative Therapies* 2000; 6(4):70–76.

Madrigal-Santillan, E, et al. "Review of natural products with hepatoprotective effects." *World Journal of Gastroenterology* 2014; 20(40):14787–14804.

Percival, M. "Nutritional Support for Detoxification." *ANSR—Applied Nutritional Science Reports* 1999. www.acudoc.com/Detoxification.PDF

Valdecantos, MP, et al. "Lipoic acid improves mitochondrial function in nonalcoholic steatosis through the stimulation of sirtuin 1 and sirtuin 3." *Obesity (Silver Spring)* 2012; 20(10): 1974–1983.

CHAPTER 9

Assy, N, et al. "Olive oil consumption and non-alcoholic fatty liver disease." *World Journal of Gastroenterology* 2009; 15(15):1809–1815.

Assy, N, et al. "Soft drink consumption linked with fatty liver in the absence of traditional risk factors." *Canadian Journal of Gastroenterology* 2008; 22(10):811–816.

Capanni, M, et al. "Prolonged n-3 polyunsaturated fatty acid supplementation ameliorates hepatic steatosis in patients with non-alcoholic fatty liver disease: a pilot study." *Alimentary Pharmacology and Therapeutics* 2006; 23(8): 1143–1151.

Charlton, M. "Branched-chain amino acid enriched supplements as therapy for liver disease." *Journal of Nutrition* 2006; 136(1 Suppl):295S–298S.

Cutler, N. "How to support your liver with balanced nutrition." *Liversupport.com.* May 4, 2006. www.liversupport.com/influencing-liver-disease-with-diet/

"Diet – liver disease." *MedlinePlus.* Last modified April 20, 2015. www.nlm.nih.gov/med lineplus/ency/article/002441.htm

"Eating tips for people with cirrhosis." *U.S. Department of Veterans Affairs.* Last modified Sep. 1, 2015. www.hepatitis.va.gov/patient/daily/diet/tips-for-people-with-cirrhosis.asp

Eghtesad, S, H Poustchi, and R Malekzadeh. "Malnutrition in liver cirrhosis: the influence of protein and sodium." *Middle East Journal of Digestive Diseases* 2013; 5(2): 65–75.

El-Din, SH, et al. "Pharmacological and antioxidant actions of garlic and/or onion in non-alcoholic fatty liver disease (NAFLD) in rats." *Journal of the Egyptian Society of Parasitology* 2014; 44(2): 295–308.

FDA. "Lowering salt in your diet." *U.S. Food and Drug Administration.* Last modified July 25, 2015. www.fda.gov/ForConsumers/ConsumerUpdates/ucm181577.htm

Freedman, ND, et al. "Association of meat and fat intake with liver disease and hepatocellular carcinoma in the NIH-AARP cohort." *Journal of the National Cancer Institute* 2010; 102(17): 1354–1365.

Gao, M, et al. "Fish consumption and n-3 polyunsaturated fatty acids, and risk of hepatocellular carcinoma: systematic review and meta-analysis." *Cancer Causes and Control* 2015; 26(3):367–376.

Greiner, AK, RV Papineni, and S Umar. "Chemoprevention in gastrointestinal physiology and disease. Natural products and microbiome." *American Journal of Physiology: Gastrointestinal and Liver Physiology* 2014; 307(1):G1–G15.

Group, E. "14 foods that cleanse the liver." *Global Healing Center.* Last modified Oct. 5, 2015. www.globalhealingcenter.com/natural-health/liver-cleanse-foods/

Kaukinen, K, et al. "Celiac disease in patients with severe liver disease: Gluten-free diet may reverse hepatic failure." *Gastroenterology* 2002; 122(4): 881–888.

Lai, HS, et al. "Effects of a high-fiber diet on hepatocyte apoptosis and liver regeneration after partial hepatectomy in rats with fatty liver." *Journal of Parenteral and Enteral Nutrition* 2005; 29(6): 401–407.

Mayo Clinic staff. "Gluten-free diet." *Mayo Clinic.* Nov. 25, 2014. www.mayoclinic.org/healthy-lifestyle/nutrition-and-healthy-eating/in-depth/gluten-free-diet/art-20048530

Nguyen, D, and T Morgan. "Protein restriction in hepatic encephalopathy is appropriate for selected patients: a point of view." *Hepatology International* 2014; 8(2):447–451.

Ryan, MC, et al. "The Mediterranean diet improves hepatic steatosis and insulin sensitivity in individuals with non-alcoholic fatty liver disease." *Journal of Hepatology* 2013; 59(1):138–143.

Sofi, F, and A Casini. "Mediterranean diet and non-alcoholic fatty liver disease: new therapeutic option around the corner?" *World Journal of Gastroenterology* 2014; 20(23):7339–7346.

Sullivan, S. "Implications of diet on nonalcoholic fatty liver disease." *Current Opinion in Gastroenterology* 2010; 26(2): 160–164.

Tsien, C, et al. "Metabolic and molecular responses to leucine-enriched branched chain amino acid supplementation in the skeletal muscle of alcoholic cirrhosis." *Hepatology* 2015; 61(6):2018–2029.

Wakim-Fleming, J, et al. "Prevalence of celiac disease in cirrhosis and outcome of cirrhosis on a gluten free diet: a prospective study." *Journal of Hepatology* 2014; 61(3): 558–563.

Yang, Y, et al. "Increased intake of vegetables, but not fruit, reduces risk for hepatocellular carcinoma: a meta-analysis." *Gastroenterology* 2014 Nov; 147(5):1031–1042.

CHAPTER 10

Abenavoli, L, et al. "Milk thistle in liver diseases: past, present, future." *Phytotherapy Research* 2010; 24(10):1423–1432.

"Acetadote (acetylcysteine) injection package insert." *U.S. Food and Drug Administration.* Feb. 15, 2006. www.accessdata.fda.gov/drugsatfda_docs/label/2006/021539s004lbl.pdf

Anggakusuma, et al. "Turmeric curcumin inhibits entry of all hepatitis C virus genotypes into human liver cells." *Gut* 2014; 63(7):1137–1149.

Baghdasaryan, A, et al. "Curcumin improves sclerosing cholangitis in Mdr2-/- mice by inhibition of cholangiocyte inflammatory response and portal myofibroblast proliferation." *Gut* 2010; 59(4): 521–530.

"Beware of products promising miracle weight loss." *U.S. Food and Drug Administration.* Last modified Jan. 5, 2015. www.fda.gov/ForConsumers/ConsumerUpdates/ucm 246742.htm

Buss, C, et al. "Probiotics and synbiotics may improve liver aminotransferases levels in non-alcoholic fatty liver disease patients." *Annals of Hepatology* 2014; 13(5):482–488.

Bustamante, J, et al. "Alpha-lipoic acid in liver metabolism and disease." *Free Radical Biology and Medicine* 1998; 24(6):1023–1039.

Chen, S, et al. "Coffee and non-alcoholic fatty liver disease: brewing evidence for hepatoprotection?" *Journal of Gastroenterology and Hepatology* 2014; 29(3): 435–441.

Cichoz-Lach, H, and A Michalak. "Oxidative stress as a crucial factor in liver disease." *World Journal of Gastroenterology* 2014; 20(25): 8082–8091.

"Comfrey." *LiverTox by National Institutes of Health.* Last modified March 24, 2016. http://livertox.nlm.nih.gov/Comfrey.htm

Flora, K, et al. "Milk thistle (Silybum marianum) for the therapy of liver disease." *The American Journal of Gastroenterology* 1998; 93(2):139–143.

"Glutathione." *WebMD.* Accessed Feb. 26, 2016. http://w ww.webmd.com/vitamins-supplements/ingredientmono-717-glutathione.aspx?activeingredientid=717

Gonciarz, M, et al. "The effects of long-term melatonin treatment on plasma liver enzymes levels and plasma concentrations of lipids and melatonin in patients with nonalcoholic steatohepatitis: a pilot study." *Journal of Physiology and Pharmacology* 2012; 63(1): 35–40.

Gonciarz, M, et al. "The pilot study of 3-month course of melatonin treatment of patients with nonalcoholic steatohepatitis: effect on plasma levels of liver enzymes, lipids and melatonin." *Journal of Physiology and Pharmacology* 2010; 61(6): 705–710.

Gratz, SW, H Mykkanen, and HS El-Nezami. "Probiotics and gut health: a special focus on liver disease." *World Journal of Gastroenterology* 2010; 16(4): 403–410.

Heller, JL, D Zieve, and I Ogilvie. "Acetaminophen overdose." *MedlinePlus.* Last modified Jan. 23, 2015. https://www.nlm.nih.gov/medlineplus/ency/article/002598.htm

Higdon, J. "Lipoic acid." *Linus Pauling Institute at Oregon State University.* Last modified Jan. 2012. http://lpi.oregonstate.edu/mic/dietary-factors/lipoic-acid

Hurwitz, BE, et al. "Suppression of human immunodeficiency virus type 1 viral load with selenium supplementation: a randomized controlled trial." *Archives of Internal Medicine* 2007; 167(2):148–154.

Jablonski, KL, et al. "Low 25-hydroxyvitamin D level is independently associated with non-alcoholic fatty liver disease." *Nutrition, Metabolism, and Cardiovascular Diseases* 2013; 23(8):792–798.

"Kava Kava." *LiverTox by National Institutes of Health.* Last modified March 24, 2016. http://livertox.nlm.nih.gov/KavaKava.htm

Kennedy, OJ, et al. "Systematic review with meta-analysis: coffee consumption and the risk of cirrhosis." *Alimentary Pharmacology & Therapeutics* 2016; 43(5): 562–574.

Kerksick, C, and D Willoughby. "The antioxidant role of glutathione and n-acetyl-cysteine supplements and exercise-induced oxidative stress." *Journal of the International Society of Sports Nutrition* 2005; 2(2): 38–44.

Khan, MS, et al. "The possible role of selenium concentration in hepatitis B and C patients." *Saudi Journal of Gastroenterology* 2012; 18(2):106–110.

Khoshbaten, M, et al. "N-acetylcysteine improves liver function in patients with non-alcoholic fatty liver disease." *Hepatitis Monthly* 2010; 10(1): 12–16.

"N-acetyl cysteine." *WebMD*. Accessed Feb. 26, 2016. www.webmd.com/vitamins-supplements/ingredientmono-1018-n-acetyl%20cysteine.aspx?activeingredientid=1018

National Cancer Institute. "Milk Thistle—Patient Version." *National Institutes of Health (NIH)*. Last modified Dec. 11, 2015. www.cancer.gov/about-cancer/treatment/cam/patient/milk-thistle-pdq

Office of Dietary Supplements. "Dietary Supplement Fact Sheets: Iron, Selenium, Vitamin A, Vitamin D, Vitamin E, Selenium." *National Institutes of Health.* Accessed Feb. 25, 2016. https://ods.od.nih.gov/factsheets/list-all/

Saad, RA, MF El-Bab, and AA Shalaby. "Attenuation of acute and chronic liver injury by melatonin in rats." *Journal of Taibah University for Science* 2013; 7(2): 88–96.

Sharma, V, S Garg, and S Aggarwal. "Probiotics and liver disease." *The Permanente Journal* 2013; 17(4): 62–67.

Sheehan, HB, et al. "High rates of serum selenium deficiency among HIV- and HCV-infected and uninfected drug users in Buenos Aires, Argentina." *Public Health Nutrition* 2012; 15(3):538–545.

Skaaby, T, et al. "Vitamin D status, liver enzymes, and incident liver disease and mortality: a general population study." *Endocrine* 2014; 47(1):213–220.

Stacchiotti, A, et al. "Hepatic macrosteatosis is partially converted to microsteatosis by melatonin supplementation in ob/ob mice non-alcoholic fatty liver disease." *PLoS One* 2016; 11(1): e0148115.

Xiao, Q, et al. "Inverse associations of total and decaffeinated coffee with liver enzyme levels in National Health and Nutrition Examination Survey 1999–2010." *Hepatology* 2014; 60(6): 2091–2098.

Xu, J, et al. "Effects of probiotic therapy on hepatic encephalopathy in patients with liver cirrhosis: an updated meta-analysis of six randomized controlled trials." *Hepatobiliary and Pancreatic Diseases International* 2014; 13(4):354–360.

Yiu, WF, et al. "Attenuation of fatty liver and prevention of hypercholesterolemia by extract of Curcuma longa through regulating the expression of CYP7A1, LDL-receptor, HO-1, and HMG-CoA reductase." *Journal of Food Science* 2011; 76(3):H80–H89.

CHAPTER 11

American Diabetes Association. "Physical activity is important." *Diabetes.org*. Last modified April 9, 2015. www.diabetes.org/food-and-fitness/fitness/physical-activity-is-important.html

Cho, J, et al. "Effect of aerobic exercise training on non-alcoholic fatty liver disease induced by a high fat diet in C57BL/6 mice." *Journal of Exercise Nutrition and Biochemistry* 2014; 18(4):339–346.

Cooke, M, et al. "Effects of acute and 14-day coenzyme Q10 supplementation on exercise performance in both trained and untrained individuals." *Journal of the International Society of Sports Nutrition* 2008; 5: 8.

Hallsworth, K, et al. "Resistance exercise reduces liver fat and its mediators in non-alcoholic fatty liver disease independent of weight loss." *Gut* 2011; 60(9): 1278–1283.

Hickman, IJ, et al. "Modest weight loss and physical activity in overweight patients with chronic liver disease results in sustained improvements in alanine aminotransferase, fasting insulin, and quality of life." *Gut* 2004; 53: 413–419.

Keating, SE, et al. "Exercise and non-alcoholic fatty liver disease: a systematic review and meta-analysis." *Journal of Hepatology* 2012; 57(1):157–166.

Kraus, WE, et al. "Effects of the amount and intensity of exercise on plasma lipoproteins." *The New England Journal of Medicine* 2002; 347: 1483–1492.

Lee, S, et al. "Effects of aerobic versus resistance exercise without caloric restriction on abdominal fat, intrahepatic lipid, and insulin sensitivity in obese adolescent boys: a randomized, controlled trial." *Diabetes* 2012; 61(11): 2787–2795.

Lohrey, J. "The effect of exercise on liver function." *LiveStrong Foundation*. Last modified Oct. 24, 2010. www.livestrong.com/article/287774-the-effect-of-exercise-on-liver-function/

Rector, RS, et al. "Daily exercise vs. caloric restriction for prevention of nonalcoholic fatty liver disease in the OLETF rat model." *American Journal of Physiology Gastrointestinal and Liver Physiology* 2011; 300(5): G874–G883.

Rosenfeldt, F, et al. "Systematic review of effect of coenzyme Q10 in physical exercise, hypertension and heart failure." *Biofactors* 2003; 18(1–4): 91–100.

Screenivasa, BC, et al. "Effect of exercise and dietary modification on serum aminotransferase levels in patients with nonalcoholic steatohepatitis." *Journal of Gastroenterology and Hepatology* 2006; 21(1 pt 1): 191–198.

Van Gammeren, D, D Falk, and J Antonio. "The effects of four weeks of ribose supplementation on body composition and exercise performance in healthy, young, male recreational bodybuilders: a double-blind, placebo-controlled trial." *Current Therapeutic Research* 2002; 63(8): 486–495.

Volek, J. "L-carnitine burns body fat, boosts recovery, reduces muscle soreness and protects the heart." *Nutrition Express*. Accessed March 9, 2016. www.nutritionexpress.com/article+index/protein/showarticle.aspx?id=1487

Volek, J, et al. "L-carnitine L-tartrate supplementation favorably affects markers of recovery from exercise stress." *American Journal of Physiology—Endocrinology and Metabolism* 2002; 282(2): E474–E482.

About the Author

Rich Snyder, DO, holds a medical degree from the Philadelphia College of Osteopathic Medicine. He completed his residency in Internal Medicine at Abington Memorial Hospital and his Nephrology Fellowship at the Hospital of the University of Pennsylvania. He is board certified in both Internal Medicine and Nephrology.

Dr. Snyder is the best-selling author of *What You Must Know About Kidney Disease* and *What You Must Know About Dialysis.* In addition to being a popular speaker, Dr. Snyder has appeared on numerous radio and televisions shows throughout North America. Currently, Dr. Snyder maintains a clinical nephrology practice in Easton, Pennsylvania.

Index